D1609099

LA FIGA

VISIONS OF FOOD AND FORM

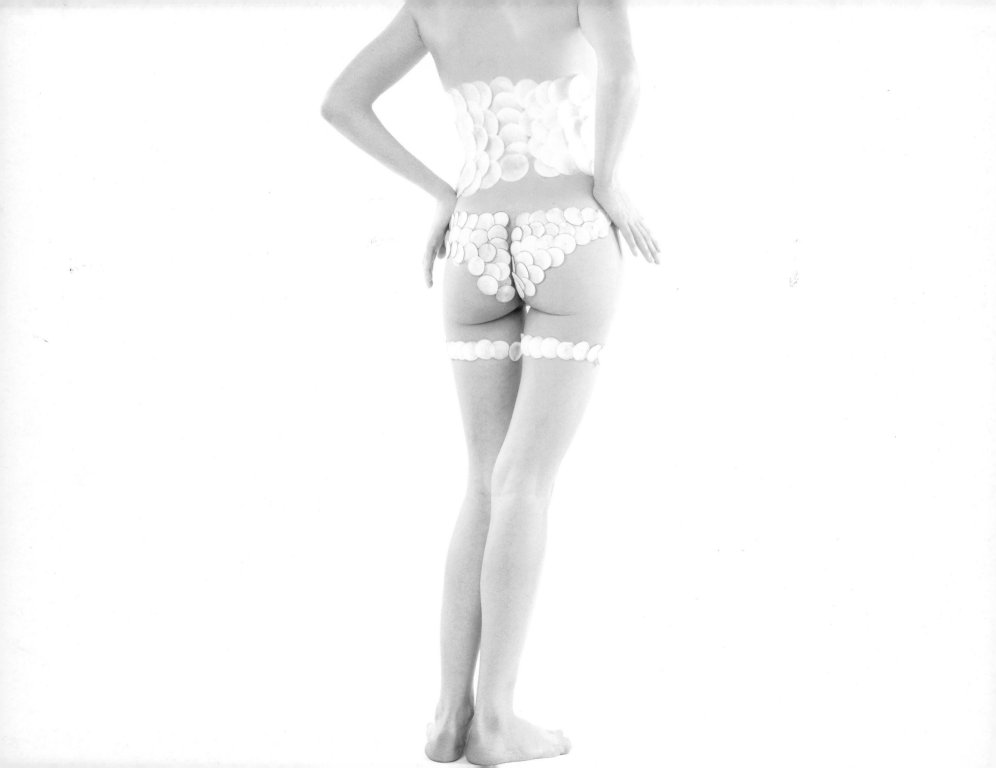

LA FIGA

VISIONS OF FOOD AND FORM

BY CHEF TIBERIO SIMONE   PHOTOGRAPHED BY MATT FREEDMAN

Published by
Book Publishers Network
P. O. Box 2256
Bothell, WA 98041
425 483-3040
www.bookpublishersnetwork.com

10 9 8 7 6 5 4 3 2 1

Printed in Canada

ISBN 10:   1-935359-75-4
ISBN 13:   978-1-935359-75-3

Edited by Lori Zue
www.LoriZueEdits.com

Designed by Phil Kovacevich

LAFIGAPROJECT.COM

CONTENTS

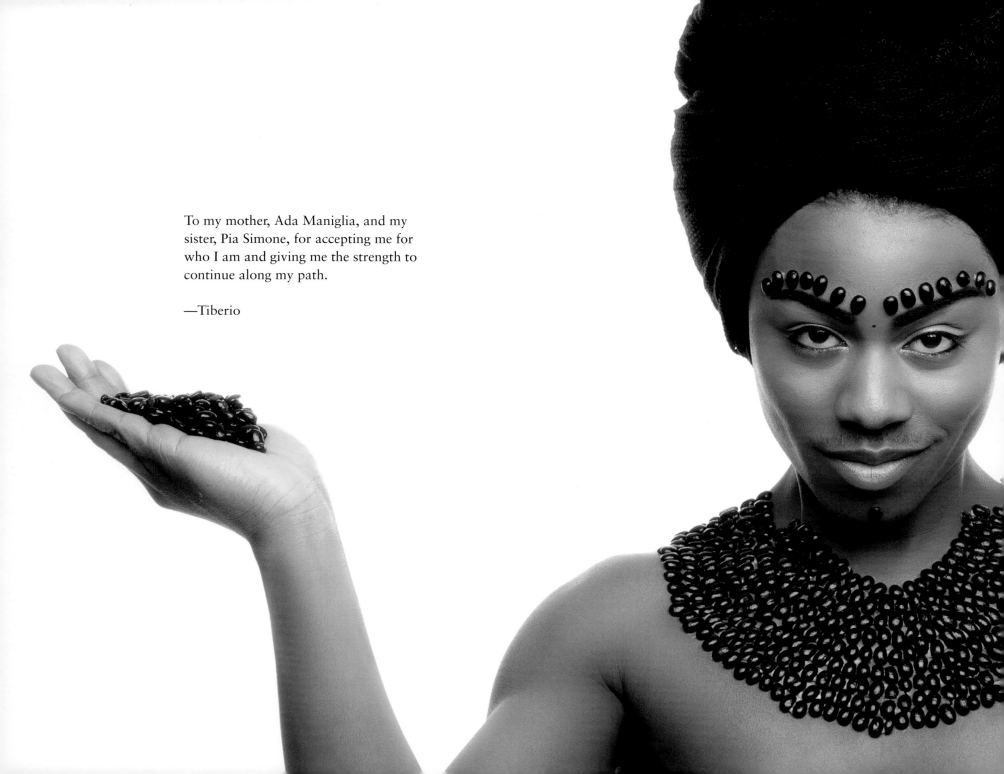

To my mother, Ada Maniglia, and my sister, Pia Simone, for accepting me for who I am and giving me the strength to continue along my path.

—Tiberio

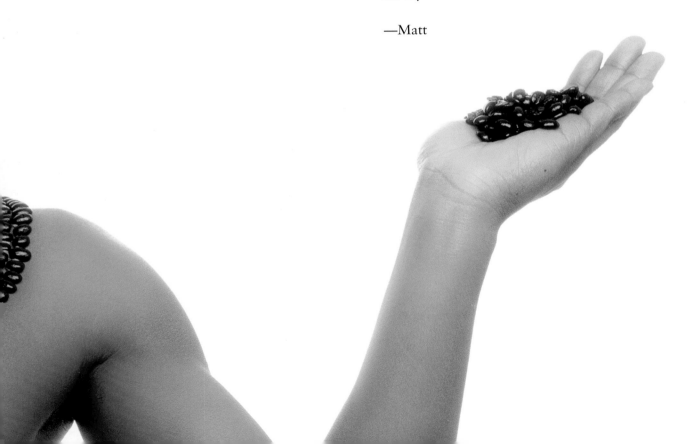

To my parents, Marilyn and Larry Freedman, for allowing me the freedom to explore and always believing in me, no matter what. And for giving me my first camera.

—Matt

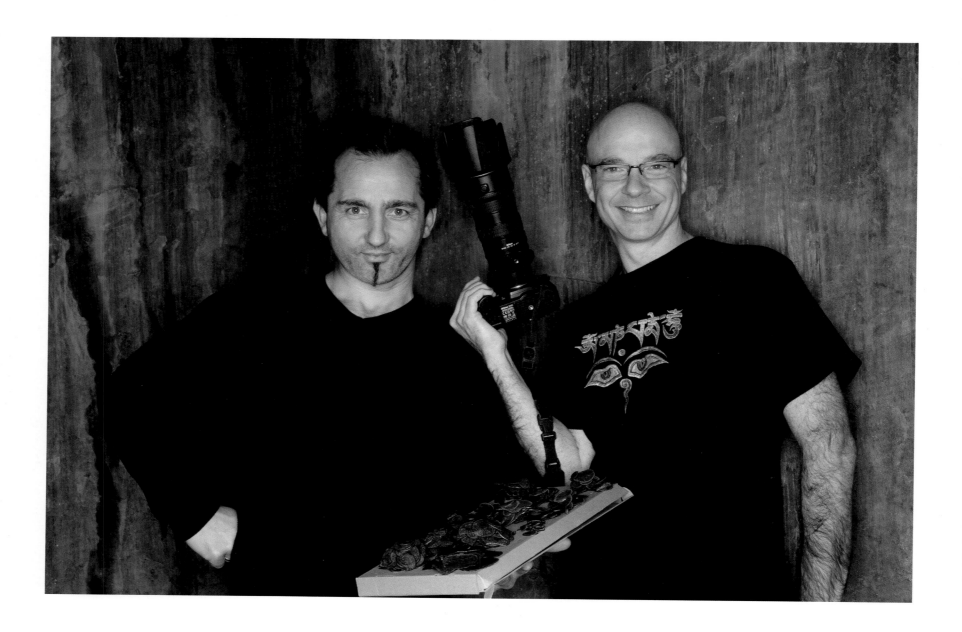

FOREWORD

MOST PEOPLE VIVIDLY REMEMBER the first time they encounter Tiberio Simone, and sometimes it seems that everyone knows Tiberio. I was at a Christmas party for entrepreneurs in Seattle, making awkward small talk around the dessert table and privately praying that the dance music would start. Tiberio, the evening's pastry chef, strutted across the room in his leather pants with unabashed Southern Italian flair. Within a few minutes, he was hand-feeding me chocolate creations as we delved into subjects ranging from love to the existential search for meaning. His vibrant, inimitable spirit was like a lightning bolt of color exploding across a gray Seattle skyline—sometimes stunning and always marvelous.

Tiberio will be the first to tell you that his love for simple but beautiful food began in his mother's Italian kitchen. Nothing can improve upon the freshest tomato grown in his garden or the mushroom he digs up during a rainy Western Washington fall. As much as this James Beard Award winner has a reputation for making beautiful cakes that delight the palate, Tiberio also provides emotional nourishment to those around him with his unique recipe of kindness, generosity, playfulness, and forthrightness. Tiberio's motto is "I love everybody, and you are next!"

Until he collaborated with photographer Matt Freedman, Tiberio's culinary creations were ephemeral. Matt's work is stunning. His portraits capture his subject's spirit and his travel photography makes you long to be in that place—to taste the food, to hear the people, to stand in the exact spot and take in the moments. Matt's sensual gaze and technical genius capture Tiberio's art as an imaginative reincarnation of the still life, a new vision of food and form. Matt makes gorgeous portraits of Tiberio's live installations—they are almost edible.

"Only those who will risk going too far can possibly know how far one can go," wrote T. S. Eliot. In *La Figa*, Tiberio and Matt transport us with their provocative and mesmerizing photographs to a place where a simple fruit, combined with the basic human form, explodes our senses—from a pomegranate bikini to rolling hills of ingredient-covered hips. I, for one, will never think of seaweed or avocado in the same way. *La Figa* invites us to pierce through mundane living and savor the basic ingredients of life.

NASSIM ASSEFI, MD
Physician and Novelist

9

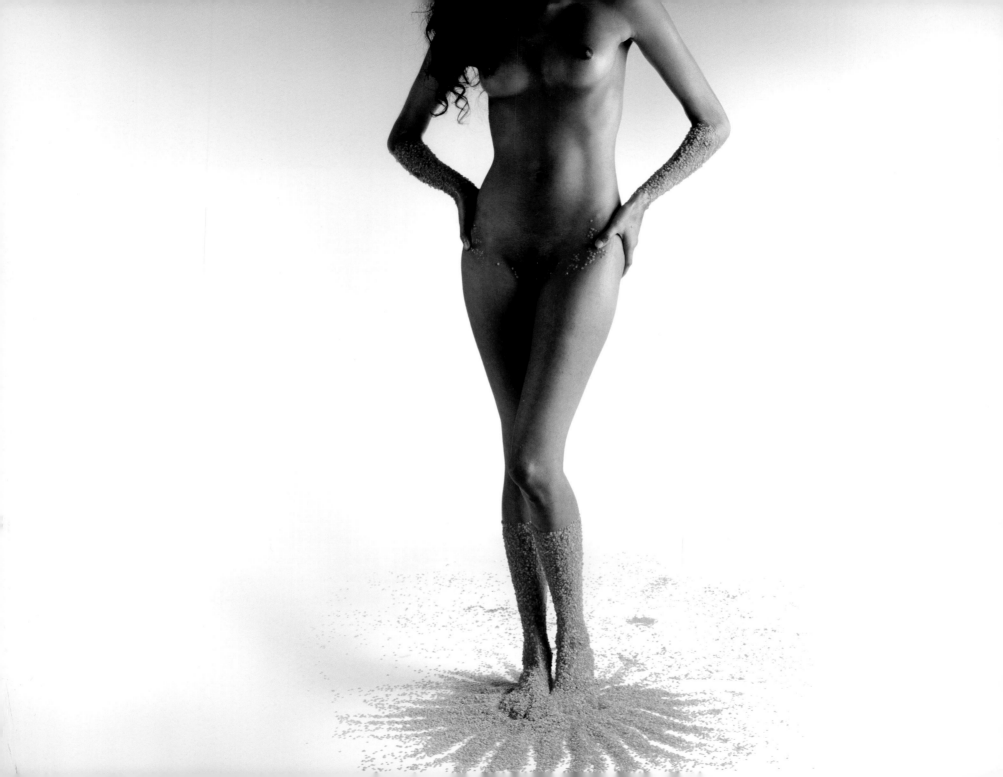

WHEN MATT AND I BEGAN THIS PROJECT in 2006, we envisioned a photography art book: a collection of thought-provoking and beautiful photographs of food art on the naked human body. Visions of food and form that hinted at the connection and relationship between the two.

We showed the early photos to friends and other people, and they asked a lot of questions. *La Figa's* message of food and touch as basic ingredients of life intrigued them. They were also intrigued by the photographs' not-so-subtle statement that good food is sensual and pleasurable—just like sex.

At that point, we began to realize that the photos weren't supposed to stand alone. People were curious about my philosophies around food, touch, and sensuality. They wanted to know how these thoughts evolved and to hear anecdotes from a lifetime of loving food.

The words in this book became my assignment. As I thought about it, I realized how much my life has been influenced by food and touch, and the healthy, natural sensuality they have in common. I began to view my life story through the lens of food: my childhood in Italy, my mother's cooking, the food I grew up with and the food I met later, the craving for a certain vegetable or fruit, my relationship with the earth and what it produces, the bounty of each season, and the memory and taste of time.

Putting these stories and recollections onto paper was an amazing feeling. It was almost like having an intimate conversation with a cherished friend. I now understand why people write and keep journals. I wish I had too, although some experiences I remember very vividly even without one. Others simply popped up as I wrote, or a smell reminded me of something from long ago. I looked forward to those memories bubbling to the surface, like little surprises. I had the privilege of reflecting on them and analyzing how those times in my life shaped the person I am now.

Someone described me as a pleasure activist. *Perfetto!* It is true; I did not know the name before, but a pleasure activist is exactly what I have been my entire life. I add more pleasure to the gourmet experience because I add sensuality. Ideally, this experience combines food and touch, but, no matter what, it will appeal to the senses and provide pleasure. I am blessed because others recognize this need in their lives and have asked me to bring my message of the sensuality of food and form to events and festivals around the world. When I received the James Beard Award for one of my desserts, I

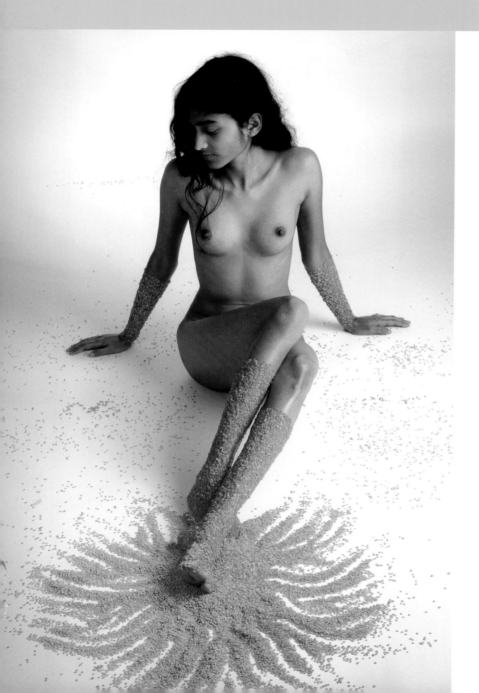

realized that even mainstream traditionalists appreciate my
belief that food should provide pleasure by activating the
senses. I feel blessed and lucky to do all the things I love and
to be rewarded in ways that bring pleasure to others, too.

If someone had told me ten years ago I would be
creating this book one day, I would never have believed it.
It is so strange how life changes and how we change with it.
Everything happens for a reason, and we need to be open to
the new paths that life presents. I am very proud of *La Figa*,
and I will continue this journey, with beauty, good food, and
sensual touch serving as my guides.

Thank you for joining me on this voyage. The images and
words in this book are meant to engage all your senses—the
same ones that are stimulated when you're served a delicious
meal or touched by someone who turns you on.

There are two things you must remember: Eat well and
make love.

Buon Appetito.

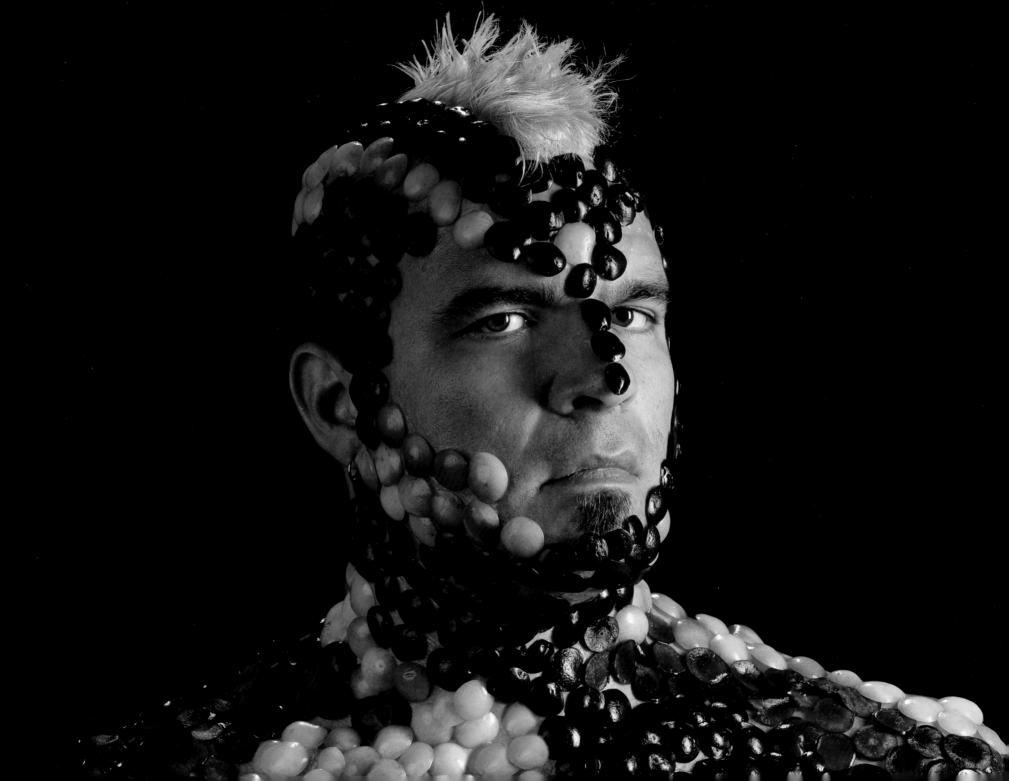

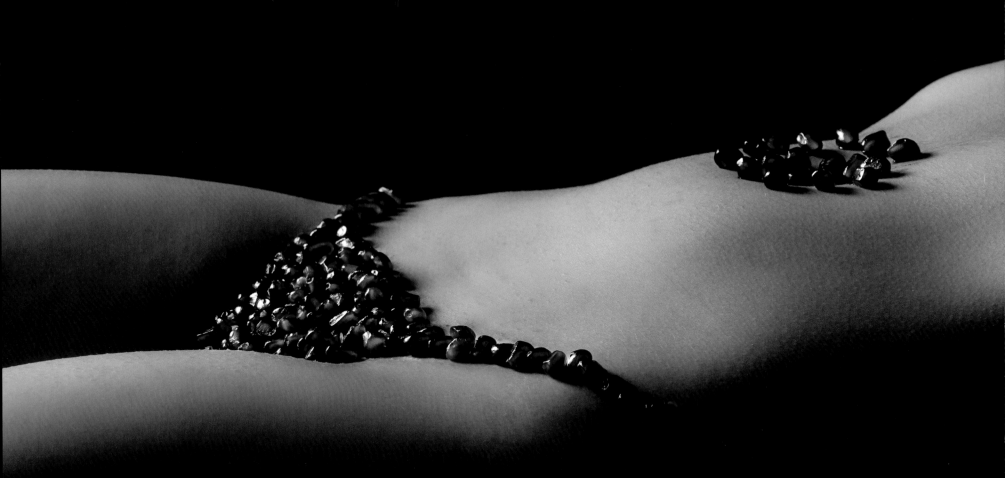

FOOD AND TOUCH

Soon after reaching adulthood, I realized that the perfect diet—the perfect *existence*—includes food and touch. Healthy, nutritious food fuels our bodies. Touching and being touched provides nutrition of a different sort, and, because of that, we can reproduce and love. Food nourishes the body from the inside out, and sex feeds it from the outside in.

SENSUALITY AND PLEASURE

Done properly, food and touch will not only provide pleasure but also engage and delight the senses. The first bite of a good meal is as promising as a first kiss. The culmination of many perfect bites is orgasmic. Food can be as sensual as sex, and both are enhanced with touch.

I love pleasure. Everybody does. Of course, pleasure comes in many forms and shapes. For me, pleasure is not just what I can get or receive, but, instead, it is more about what I can give. To live a life full of pleasure, however, we need to both give and receive it.

This book celebrates food and touch in a very elemental way. The food in the photographs is fresh, simple, and beautiful—as it was in nature. The touch of the food on the models' skin is sensuous, natural, nutritious, and life-giving.

My goal in presenting the food on the naked human body has evolved beyond art, beyond that initial concept years ago. Instead, these photographs demonstrate the fundamental fusion of food and touch, the two basic ingredients of life, with sensuality and pleasure, the two elements which give beauty and fullness to life.

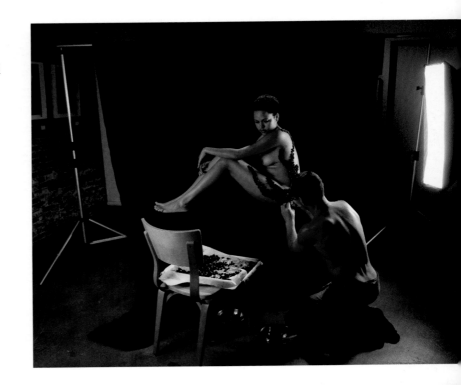

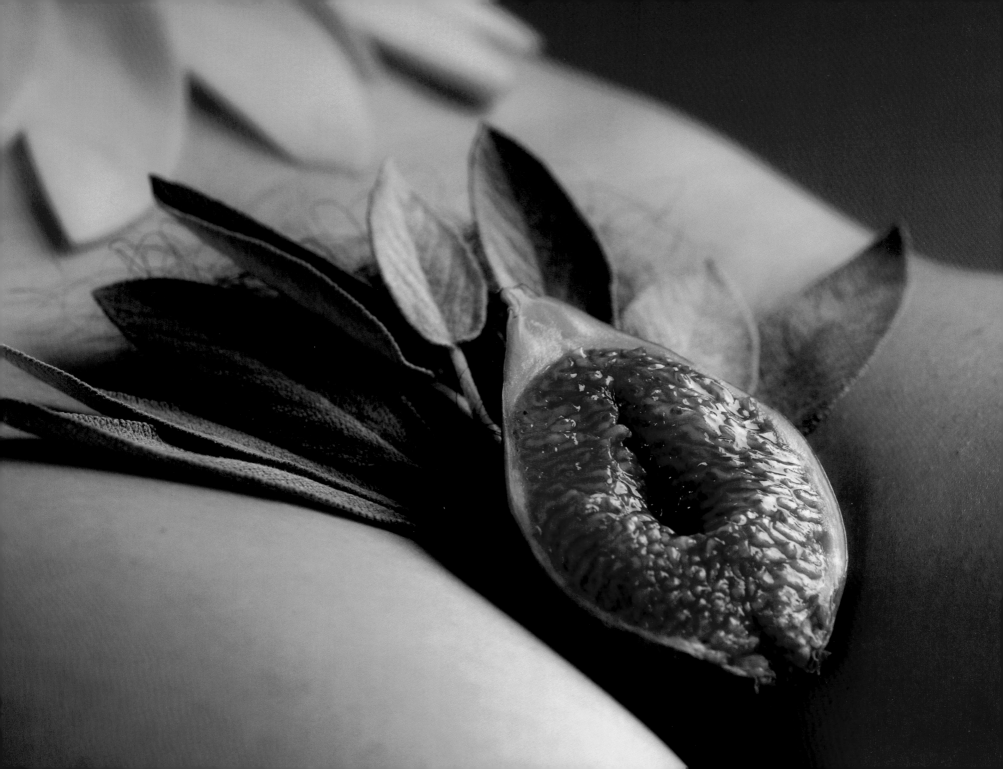

AS SOON AS I THOUGHT OF IT, the name *La Figa* was the obvious choice for my catering business and, later, for this book. As it turned out, my decision was both controversial and provocative. I shrug and laugh at the first and joyfully embrace the second.

In Italian, *la fica* refers to a fruit: the fig. *La figa* refers to a beautiful, sexy woman. *Che bella figa* means "what a lovely woman!" Since the pronunciation and spelling are so similar to the English word "fig," and I based my business in America, I used the "g" instead of a "c" and settled on *La Figa* for the name of my business. So far, so good, right? Nothing here that's offensive…or so I thought.

In fact, the name *La Figa* was perfect: My roots are intertwined with those of this fruit in Southern Italy. The fig embodies my love for the land and for its fig trees, which I've always believed produce the most wonderful fruit in the universe. Most importantly, the name *La Figa* inspires images of freshness and beauty—whether it's the fig itself or a gorgeous woman we're complimenting by likening her to this popular fruit.

Pleased I'd found a name that celebrated not only my favorite fruit but also paid homage to women, I processed the paperwork for my new business, La Figa Catering. Soon, I handed out my new business cards—with the company name and a delicious-looking picture of an open fig—to friends, including my Italian friends.

They laughed and laughed when they saw the business cards and teased me for weeks. Did I do this on purpose, they wondered. Did I name my business after the Italian word for a woman's vagina, and did I choose a picture of a fig that looks startlingly like this part of a woman's body?

This word—*la figa*—had more power and meaning than I'd originally given it credit. Certainly, I knew *la figa* referred to a beautiful woman, and of course I knew it can also mean the vagina. But I never believed (as some Italians do) this was a derogatory term for the female genitalia—or that it would be a problem for my new business's name.

My friends told me otherwise and encouraged me to change the name so potential clients wouldn't be offended. I considered their suggestion, but I just couldn't do it. I loved the name, I loved the fruit, I loved the connection to my homeland, and I loved the fact that *che bella figa* is a compliment to a beautiful and sexy woman. I still do.

Then it dawned on me: Since when is the female genitalia a bad thing? For God's sake, why *not* name the vagina after a wonderfully tasty, juicy fruit? How could that possibly be a bad thing?

Screw the people insulted by the expression, I thought.

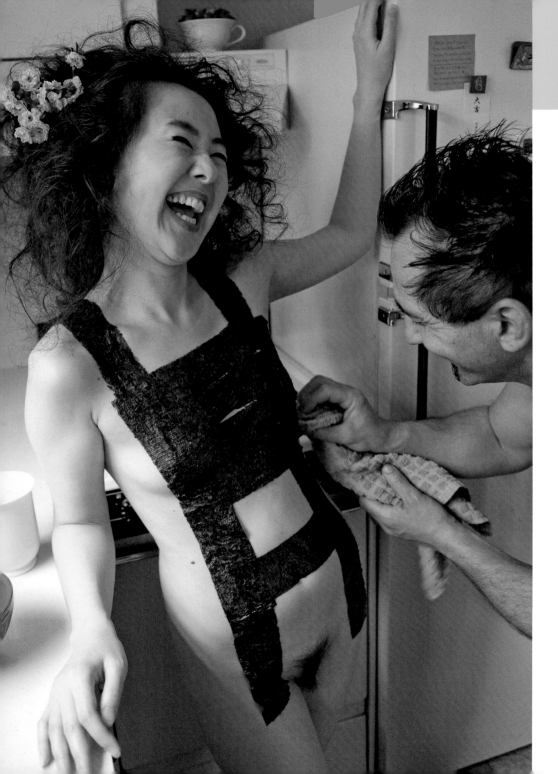

If I were a woman, I would be pleased if someone called me *la figa*—perhaps even *la figa d'oro*, which is a golden fig with amber-colored flesh.

In my opinion, *bella figa* is the highest compliment a man can give a woman. A lot of Italian men feel this way too. Many women are proud to hear the words *bella figa*, because a man usually speaks them only when he finds a woman truly attractive.

While not everyone agrees, the female genitalia connotation of *la figa* is a positive thing. Vaginas are part of the birth process; they provide amazing sexual pleasure; and many people find them pretty and fascinating. They deserve a good name. *La figa* is not derogatory toward women—it celebrates them.

I must confess, I love it when all these good meanings of *la figa* come together. Literally. If I find a woman attractive and she is interested in me, I might eat a fig directly from her genitalia—or maybe her mouth, while we get to know each other better if she is a little bit shy.

More than eight years later, I know *La Figa* is still the best possible name for my business and my book, despite its controversial and provocative meanings. And also because of them.

SINCE WHEN IS THE FEMALE GENITALIA
A BAD THING? FOR GOD'S SAKE, WHY NOT
NAME THE VAGINA AFTER A WONDERFULLY
TASTY, JUICY FRUIT?

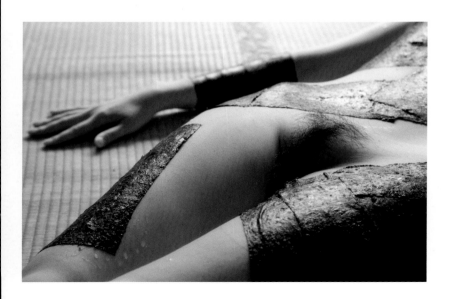

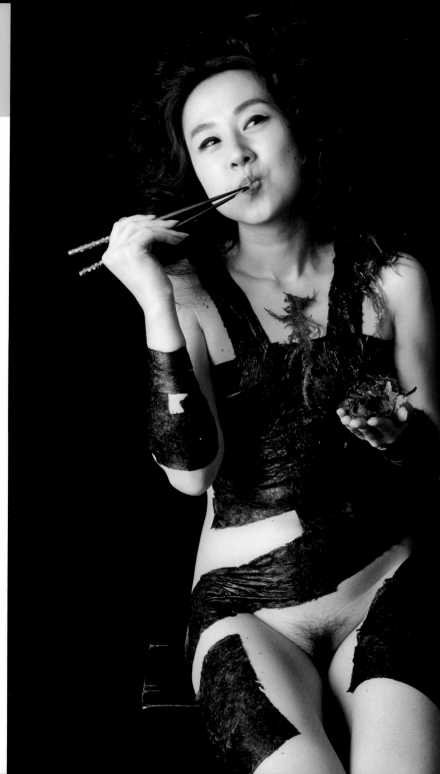

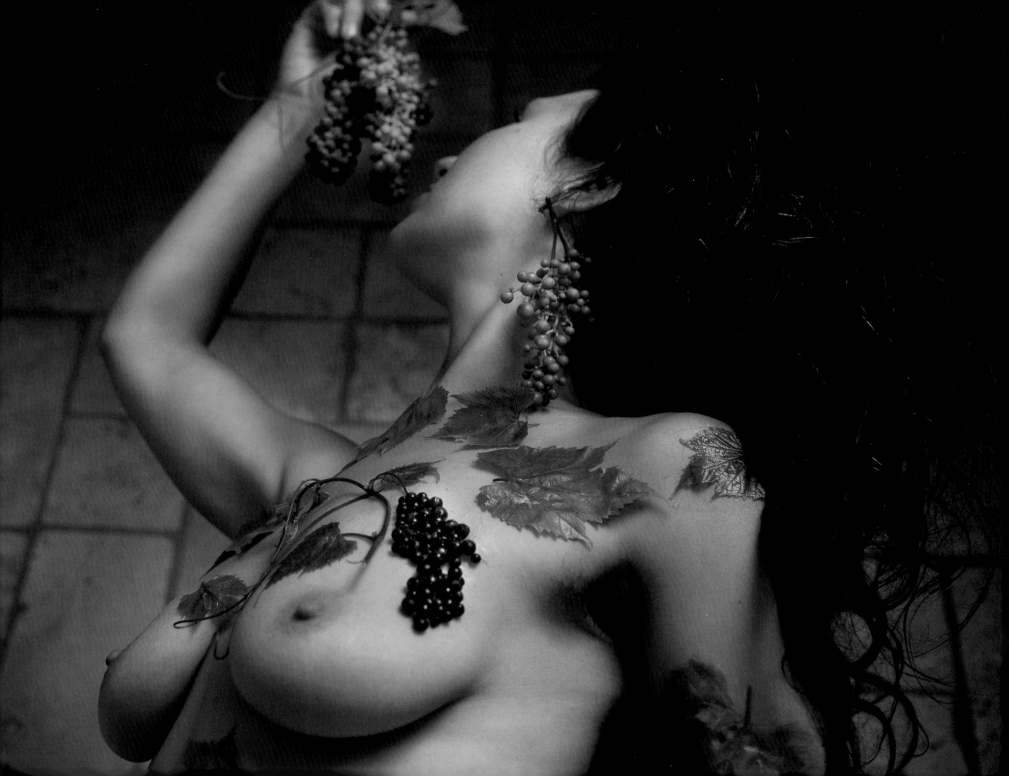

LOVE FOR FOOD

WHO DOES NOT LOVE FOOD? It is hard for me to imagine someone might feel this way because food has always been my favorite thing in the world. Truly. Even when I was a little boy, there were times when my mother had to hide anything edible because I devoured whatever I could get my hands on. I didn't learn her lessons about appreciating quality over quantity until much later; I simply craved the pleasurable experience of eating. Today, I always choose quality because I've learned this is where true pleasure lies.

Not surprisingly, my earliest memories are of food and being fed simple, wholesome ingredients which tasted like heaven to a three-year-old boy. At breakfast, my mother sat my two brothers and me next to each other on the kitchen table, held a bowl in her hand, and used a single spoon to feed each of us in turn. Our breakfast consisted of bread soaked with goat's milk and flavored with coffee and sugar. When it was my turn, my mother made sure the spoon was always a little more full, perhaps because I ate faster than anyone else, but certainly because she knew how much I appreciated and valued food. That homemade cereal tasted so incredible that whenever I go home to Italy, I eat the same thing at my mother's kitchen table.

I was a lucky boy to have a mother like mine. Despite small children underfoot and unending chores, she was an outstanding cook and worked very hard to create amazing meals using only fresh ingredients from the farm. My dad was a very stingy person; he seldom gave any money to my mom, so she rarely bought anything from the store.

I hated this situation. I almost never tasted the store-bought foods my classmates always seemed to have: prosciutto, fresh mozzarella, mortadella, and Nutella, a chocolate and hazelnut spread. These weren't part of my life. I brought the same thing to school every day: homemade bread with tomato, olive oil, and arugula—sometimes with provolone cheese (but only occasionally). Everyone else brought fancy sandwiches with all sorts of yummy ingredients from the store. I remember salivating over their food, then being embarrassed, so I hid and ate my food without being seen. I grew up with constant food cravings.

Once in a great while, my mother bought Nutella. She put only a small amount on my sandwich, probably to make the jar last longer, and that frustrated me—all it did was whet my appetite and make me realize how much I was missing out on. Sometimes, if I was lucky, I found the hidden jar of Nutella and devoured the whole thing. I couldn't stop myself—even though I knew I would get a stomachache if I ate it all…which I always did.

I took my time scooping out this chocolate heaven with my finger and placing it lovingly in my mouth. I worshipped every drop of it. As the amount of Nutella in the jar dwindled, I took smaller and smaller amounts to make it last longer. When not a lick of Nutella remained in the jar, it looked as though it had been washed with water—I was that much of an expert at getting every last morsel with my finger. I still remember the intense pleasure I got from this special treat. It was so overwhelming that I cried, but I didn't understand why I had tears when this food made me so happy.

Every time my mother found out what I had done, she chased me and yelled at the top of her lungs. I knew it was wrong, and I felt bad about it, but not bad enough to stop me from doing it again and again, and not just with Nutella, either, but with any food that we rarely had in the house or that tempted me for some reason. It was like a drug to me, so when I received a beating or other punishment for sneaking this food, I didn't care. The forbidden food was always worth it.

My dad insisted I work on the farm as a child. I never liked it, especially in the winter when we had to pick olives. It was so cold and sometimes very wet—there were times I couldn't even move my hands. I tried to find excuses to stay home because I much preferred helping my mom cook in the kitchen.

One of my best techniques was pretending I had a terrible stomachache. Even then, I used food to my advantage. My plan was detailed and genius: I chewed some bread, mixed it with bites of carrots and celery, then took a big mouthful of milk. I acted the part, forcing myself to vomit this disgusting mixture in the backyard in front of my dad. My dad could not have cared less and still insisted I work, but my mother's arguments occasionally swayed him. I think she knew I was pretending, but we never talked about it.

I could sit still for hours and watch her cook, especially when she made bread—a lengthy process that started early in the morning. I also loved watching her make pastry cream, partly because she gave me the pan and the wooden spoon when she was done, knowing I would clean every speck of cream with my tongue.

My love for food was nurtured in other ways too. I remember waiting for each season's fruits and vegetables to ripen so we could enjoy a new selection of delicious flavors. In winter, for example, the oranges and mandarins ripened, oh, so slowly as the colors on the fruit trees gradually changed from green to yellow and then finally to orange. When we could at last pick them, I always ate so many that I got sick—which never really bothered me, since I always did it again the next year, or the next season, with another fruit or vegetable. Like with the Nutella, the pleasure of eating the food I craved was worth just about anything.

I am proud and not at all surprised that I became a chef,

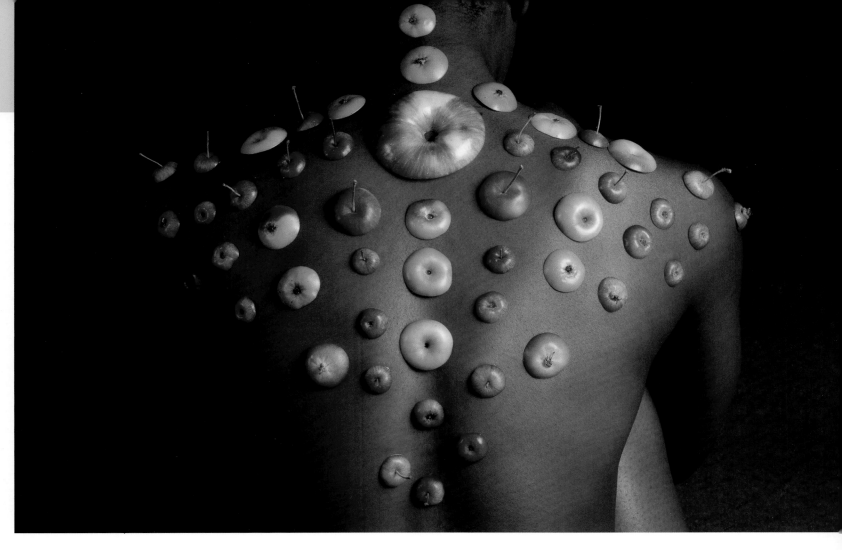

especially one whose primary pleasure comes from cooking for people and making them smile. I learned on the farm that food is a gift from nature, and I have great reverence and respect for the ingredients we use to nourish and fuel our bodies. I recognize how fortunate I am to have both quantity and quality, so I work hard to never waste anything edible and to prepare every bite with as much attention, innovation, and love as my mother did.

The way I see it: Food is love. Food is pleasure. Food is everything.

My genuine love for food will never end. It is in my roots, in my soul, in nearly every childhood memory. Food has given me so much: Life. Pleasure. Culture. A career. Friends. Lovers. Everything I am is due to food and some luck.

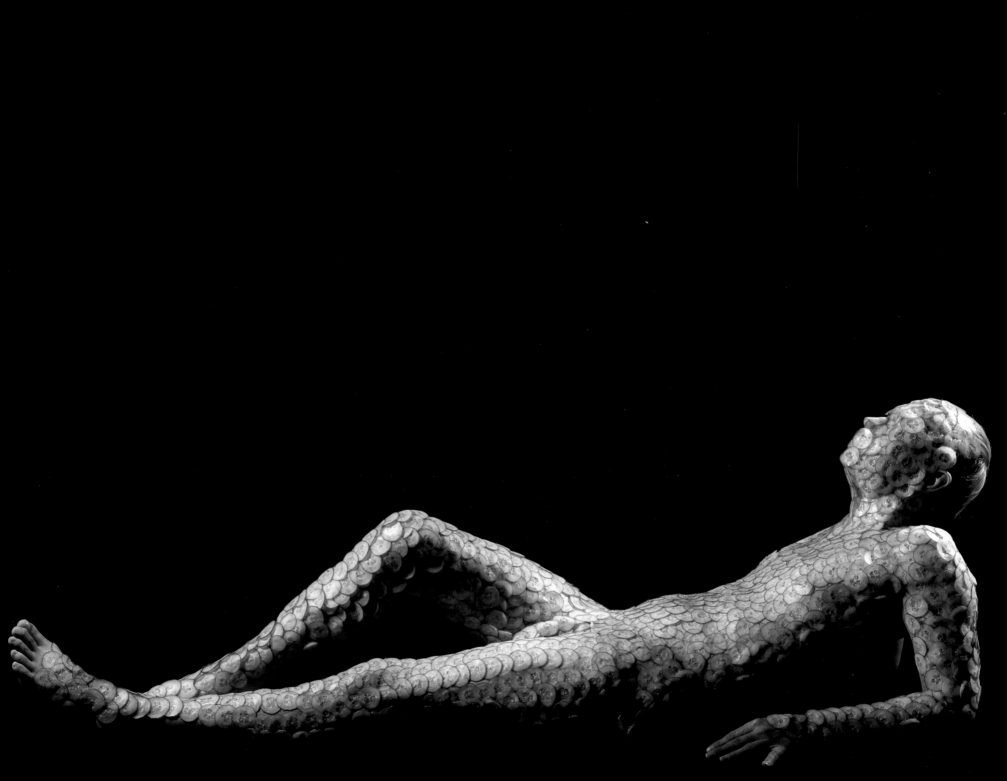

AN EXPLOSION OF JOY

I GREW UP WORKING THE LAND in Southern Italy. Those days are forever etched in my mind, and they shape my philosophy of food and life. Revisiting the stories of all the different fruits and vegetables that were part of my childhood is like spending time with friends I have loved for a lifetime.

My brothers and I were responsible for working the land with our father. In the Apulia region of Italy, an independent farmer did not work only one plot of land; our work was scattered throughout the region. The land was separated into different parcels—some big and some small—with such names as *La Cicula, Lu Patru, Lu Mea, Bandiellu, Donna Laura, La Patula, Santu Nicola,* and *Tura Noa,* from old civilizations in the area. A parcel's size was based on the type of produce that could be cultivated in that particular terrain. Because the topography was varied, our region grew many different food items, including vegetables, fruits, wheat, and tobacco. We also had quite a few orchards of olive trees, and we were known for our vineyards of Niuru Maru grapes used to make Negro Maro, a very, very dark wine with a deep, full body. We grew table grapes too, and other types for lighter wines.

Every morning, my mom packed food for us to bring to the farm and eat during the lunch break. The springtime lunches were most memorable to me because she placed in a plastic bag a few slices of bread, a good amount of cured olives, and sometimes sardo cheese, a sharply flavored hard cheese made from sheep's milk and aged for up to a year. All that was missing were vegetables, and we picked those ourselves from whichever land we were working on at the time. If that particular lot did not have vegetables, we went to the neighboring land and picked some.

All that fresh air and exercise meant I could not wait for lunch.

As I worked, I fantasized about tearing into the bread and stuffing my mouth with vegetables and olives. When we worked in the fields, I was particularly excited when the cucumbers were ripe and ready to be harvested because they were refreshing and sweet on super hot days. We weren't allowed to pick cucumbers unless they were big enough to be harvested, so when Dad gave us permission to pick some for lunch, even before he had finished his sentence, we were off and running like crazy to find the biggest cucumber. Sometimes we fought over one, which always tasted better when flavored with a win.

Without a doubt, lunch was the best part of the day. We all had our own style of eating, and my system was designed to maximize pleasure and enhance the sensual experience of eating food I'd just picked in the warm sunshine. First, I took a big bite of the cucumber, as if I was eating a banana, and chewed it slightly. Then, I took a smaller bite of bread and, halfway through chewing it and the cucumber, I added a couple of salted, cured dark olives. I used my tongue and teeth to locate all the olive pits, then spat them out, and added a tiny bit of sharp cheese to my mouth. I tried to chew this delicious combination as long as possible so the flavors would last and I could create the ultimate, heavenly taste sensation in my mouth. Mmm. Soooooo good.

Sometimes, while I was eating, my dad would ask, "Why do you close your eyes when you eat?"

Before I could swallow and reply, one of my brothers would invariably say, "Because he thinks he's eating a penis."

Then the fight would start.

To this day, I consider this very simple food to be among the most delicious I have ever eaten. For years, I wondered why, and I finally figured it out: The food was like an orgasm. On those cucumber farm days, I was working very hard, I was starving, and I desperately needed the food to give me energy to do this backbreaking work. When I finally got to eat lunch and the food arrived in my stomach, it was an explosion of joy inside of me—just like an orgasm. Chewing the food, moving it around in my mouth, savoring the flavors—these were all sensual movements and experiences leading up to that moment when I finally swallowed and shot that heavenly concoction straight into my open, needy stomach.

I wasn't the only child who enjoyed cucumbers when we were growing up; we all used them as a source of entertainment too. More times than I can remember, my brothers, my friends, and I got up in the middle of the night and sneaked out of the house. We met in a special place and often waited as long as thirty minutes for all the "Warriors of the Night" to arrive. We saw ourselves as brave soldiers who weren't afraid of anything, and we demonstrated this with stealthy visits to local farms to steal and eat whatever was in season.

One of those fun vegetables was the cucumber. We rolled around, laughing hysterically, as we stuffed cucumbers in our pants and pretended to be big men seducing women. We chased each other and acted as if we were having sex from behind.

Thinking about it now, it seems so ridiculous, but it was really good, innocent fun. I have no regrets. If I could do it all over again, I would. We felt powerful, and we enjoyed ourselves.

So, even as children, we realized the cucumber's shape resembled a penis, and we saw the vegetable as a sexual image. I have known people who have used it as a sexual toy, and they've said it can be very pleasurable. But a word of advice: Select a cucumber that is a little soft and pliable. Those fresh, crispy ones might break, creating a challenging—and very embarrassing—situation.

Have fun no matter how you seek pleasure from your cucumber. Even if, to be on the safe side, you choose to get your cucumber thrills indirectly, perhaps from the cucumber salad recipe in this book, compliments of my mother. And me.

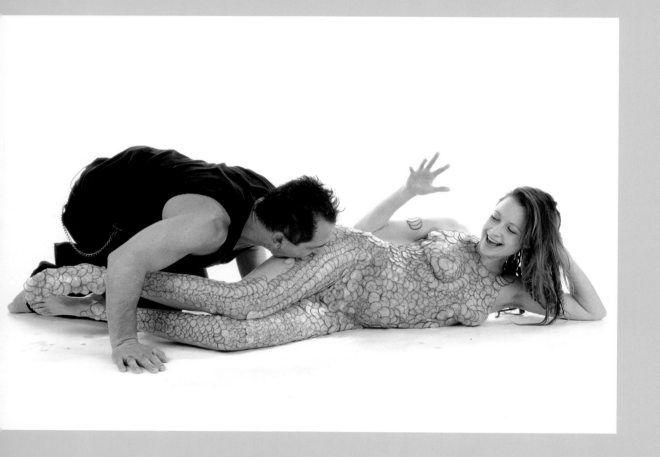
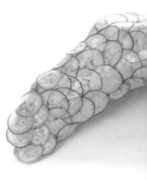

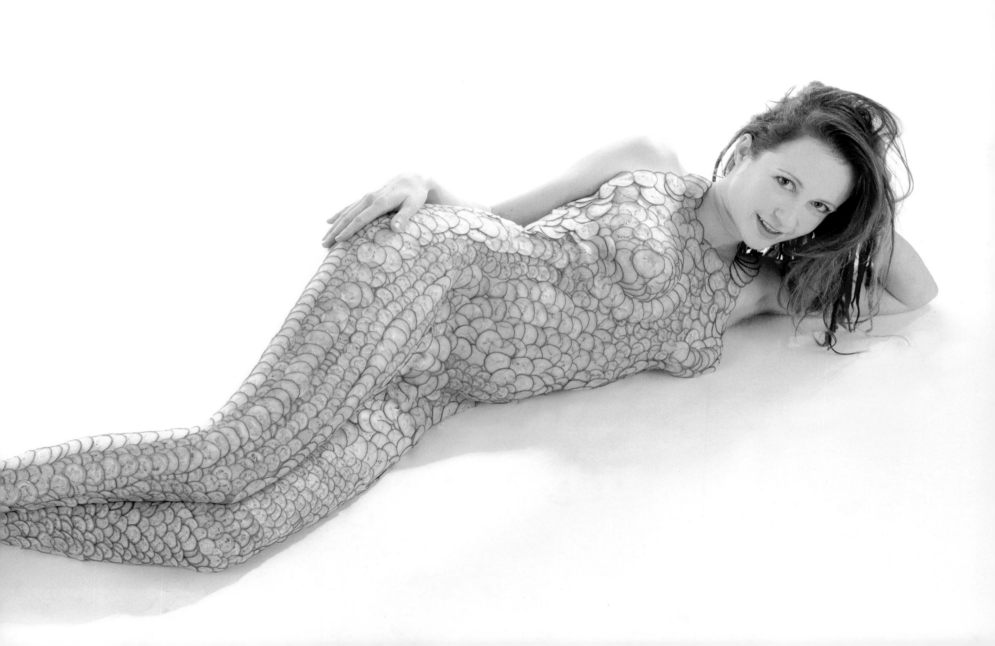

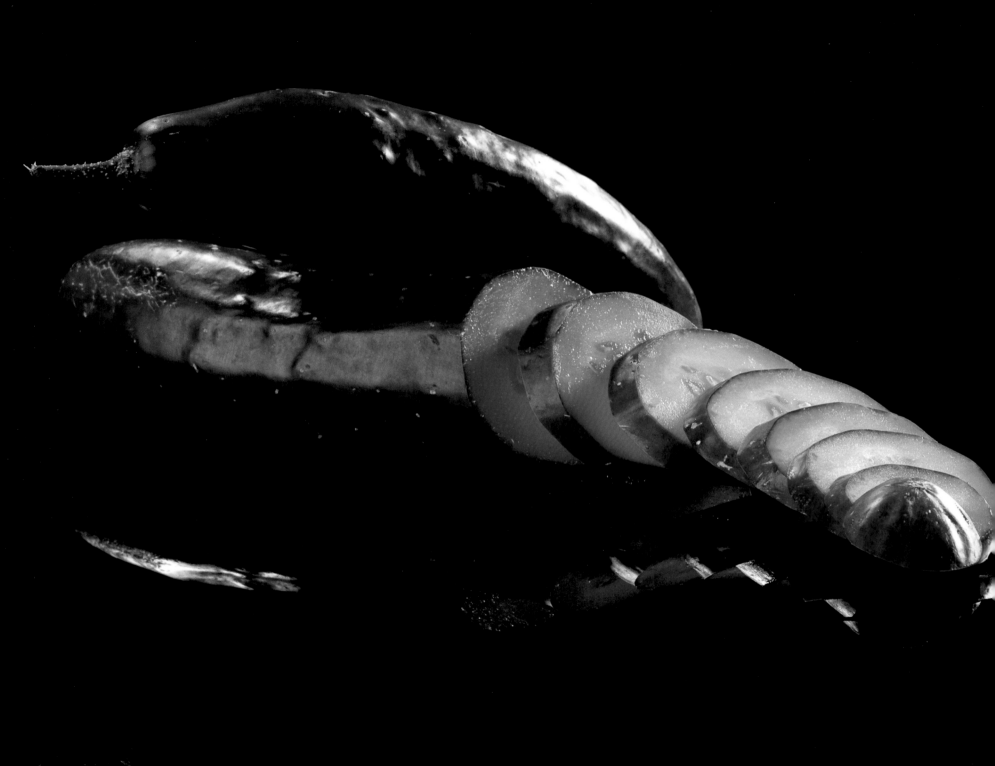

CUCUMBERS

As a child, the cucumber was a welcome sight on my dinner table. One of my favorite dishes was this cucumber salad my mother made.

When you're shopping for cucumbers, choose one that is hard and crispy. The English cucumber is delicious and not too hard to find, although when I'm in Italy, I usually prefer *le manucheddre*, which are small and stubby.

CUCUMBER SALAD

PEEL THE SKIN of several cucumbers and slice them into rounds about 1/8-inch thick. Place them in a glass serving bowl and add some red wine vinegar (depending on how strong it is) and then add some olive oil and sea salt.

Let it rest for an hour while the salt releases the water from the cucumbers. The water will mix with the other flavors and create my favorite juice for dipping bread, so be sure to serve bread with this salad.

Oh, Mamma mia, this is such a great salad. Simple. Delicious. Perfect. The natural flavors are allowed to shine, and I can taste the bounty of the earth. There's something very comforting about the subtlety of the ingredients coupled with the tartness of the red wine vinegar—a balance that tells me all is right in my world.

I actually use this recipe all the time in my catering business. It is a refreshing break from the more complex dishes. No matter when or where I make it, I am always reminded of my mom and the sun of the Italian south.

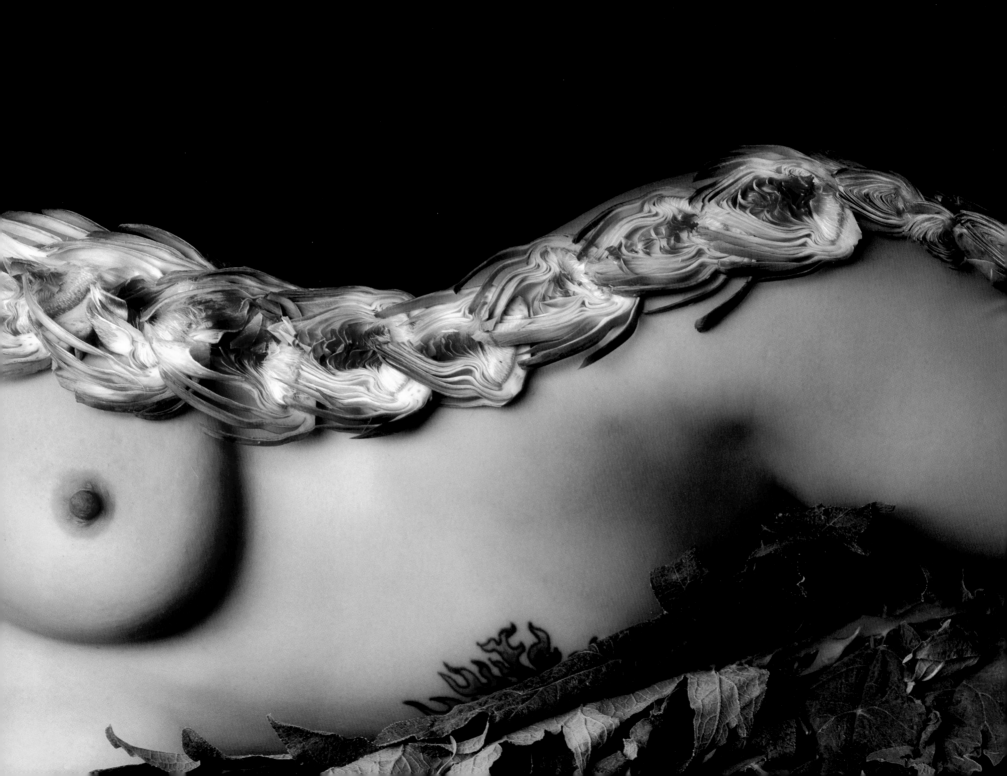

LOVE FOR TOUCH

THE FULL DIET

WHEN I THINK OF LOVE, I think of touch: hugs, a soft touch, the power of touch, making love, giving birth, a mother's touch. Touch someone's heart. Keep in touch. I feel your love. I love how you feel. Touch someone deeply. I love your touch.

Love and touch are inseparable. When we care about a person, we usually touch him or her in some way—even a simple hug or a pat on the back. Touch shows we care. The benefits of touching go both ways.

As I worked on this book, I realized how important touch is in our lives. Truly, there are only two things we need—food and touch—in order to have a full, robust life that is rich in what really matters to each of us.

I call this the full and perfect diet. Food and touch are equally important and mandatory for the art of living well. They provide good health for the body and mind.

If a baby is deprived of a mother's touch, the baby will likely struggle with emotional issues. The same is true in the animal kingdom, when young animals are separated from the mother's care.

I think we see the same effect on adults who don't receive enough touch in their lives. When people lack touch for a period of time, I believe some form of anger develops. The body does not function and it does not dance the way it would if touch was present.

Touch, and more specifically sex, is important to feed the body from the outside in. I look around at my friends, acquaintances, and even strangers, and I can sense who is being touched and who is not. You can too. The boss who is in a good mood or the teacher who is mean—our subconscious knows who has softness, touch, or sex in their lives, and who doesn't. I bet when you see a person who is happy, there is a good chance that person has sex or experiences touch in healthy, positive ways on a regular basis. There are certainly cases where people are happy despite not having sex—I believe that's possible—but only if they have a lot of love and other types of emotional touch or passion in their lives.

Children usually receive plenty of hugs, kisses, and cuddling—they thrive on it. As we get older, however, we receive less and less of it—until we meet that special someone. Then, we touch and are being touched all the time. The

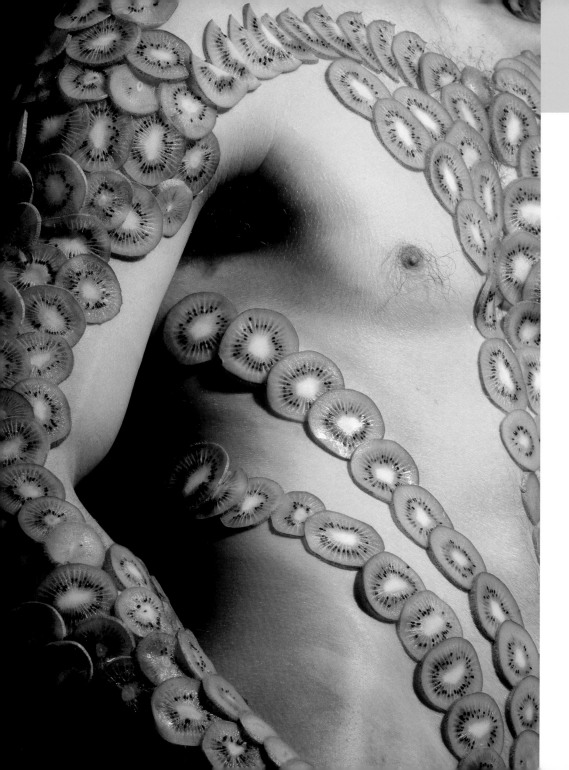

touch is now sensuous and pleasurable in ways we've never experienced.

We crave touch, just as we sometimes crave food. Bad touch is unhealthy, just as bad food makes us sick.

Most of the time, however, I believe our society lacks healthy touch. We talk about it and use "touchy-feely" words in our communication with each other, and we *want* touch… we just don't always know how to get it—or give it.

I know many sex workers whose job is to touch men— not just single men but married men who no longer have sex or touch chemistry with their partners. We have restaurants where people can go when they're hungry, so maybe we should have a restaurant where people can go for touch. They are both critical to our well-being as individuals and as a society.

I personally make sure I get the touch I need on a regular basis, and I hope I always will.

Food and touch, sensuality and pleasure—this full diet includes the essential ingredients of life. I invite you to sample from this full diet and see how quickly you appreciate and embrace a love for touch and a love for food.

Join me!

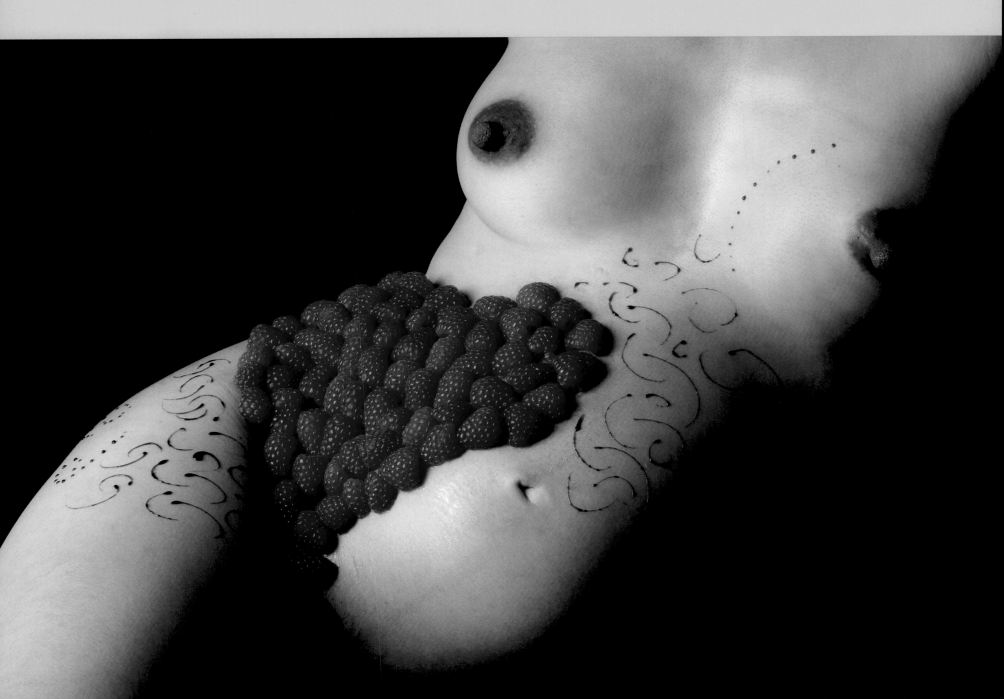

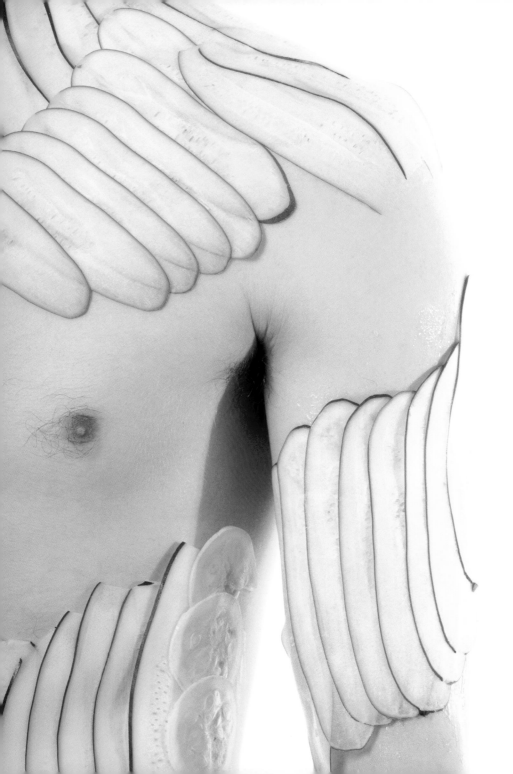

ZUCCHINI

THE ZUCCHINI was not my favorite vegetable to eat as a child; it was much more fun to play with, especially when I was about seven years old. On several occasions, a friend and I sneaked over to a neighboring farm, stole a couple zucchinis, and put them in our pants. Strutting around as if we were exceptionally well-endowed, we laughed hysterically and chased each other to a busy intersection. There, we stood nonchalantly on the corner, rolled cigarettes, and stared at everybody—hoping they would be impressed with the large protuberances jutting from the front of our pants and believe them to be real.

My love for eating zucchini finally emerged when I worked for my first professional chef, an older woman from Naples, Italy. She was an amazing chef and crazy too, in a good way. She prepared zucchini so wonderfully I felt compelled to steal again—not her zucchini, but her recipe and her technique. I've since realized she knew I was spying on her, but she was fun and allowed me this thrill.

Twenty years later, I share this recipe with you in the hope that you will try this dish and prepare it for others at your next potluck or make it for your special person to enjoy.

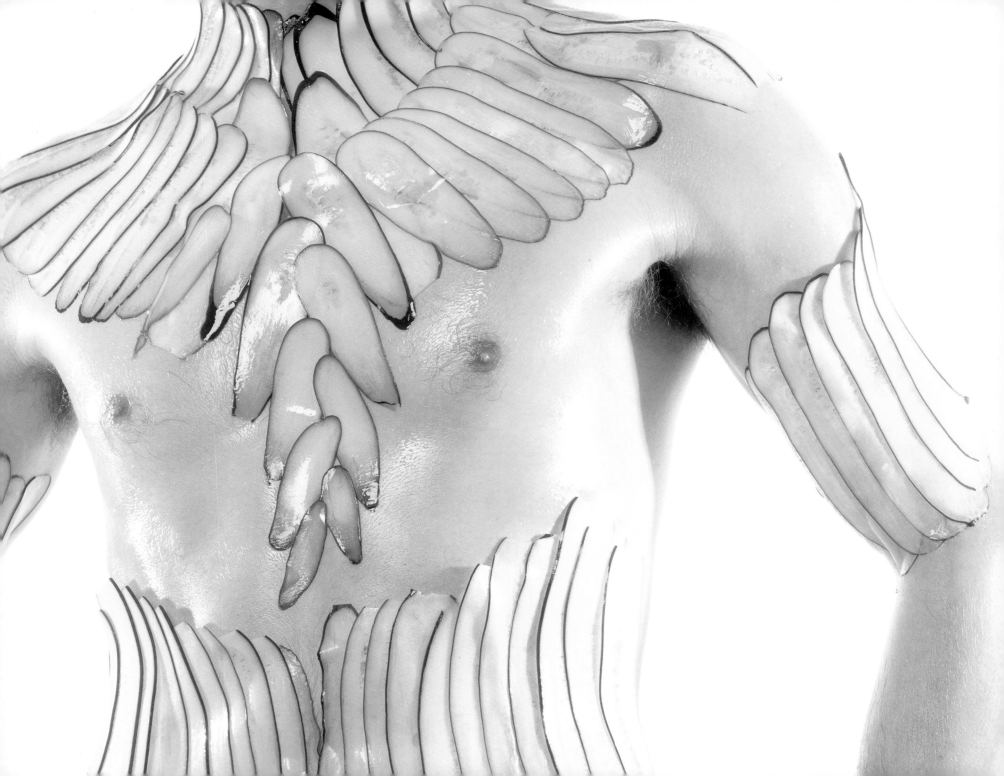

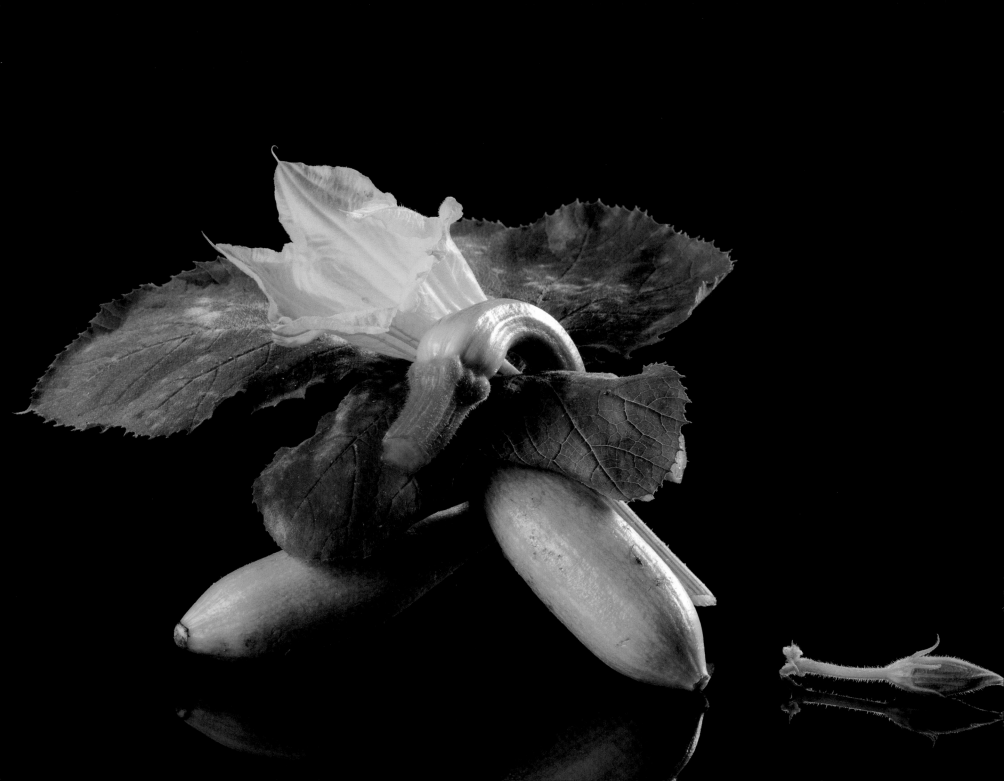

MINTED ZUCCHINI

In a bowl, whisk 2 eggs. Set them aside. In a flat dish, place a handful of flour seasoned with a teaspoon of salt and a teaspoon of black pepper. In a second flat dish, add 1 cup of bread crumbs mixed with 1/3 cup of pecorino romano cheese.

Slice a zucchini lengthwise into 1/3-inch strips. Fold the slices into the flour and shake off the extra flour, then dip the zucchini in the egg mixture, making sure every surface is coated with egg. Next, fold the zucchini in the bread crumb and cheese mixture. Press down—but not too hard—with the palm of your hand so plenty of the bread mixture sticks to and covers all the surfaces of the strips. This makes for a thicker crust and firmer texture.

Fry the zucchini strips in hot oil until they are golden brown on both sides. Place them on a parchment-paper-lined baking sheet to cool and to absorb the extra oil.

In a small bowl, combine the chopped pieces of 15 leaves of fresh mint, 1 cup of good olive oil, 1/4 cup of balsamic vinegar, about 1 teaspoon of salt, and a teaspoon of dried red chili pepper. Mix these ingredients well to create the dressing.

Wait until the fried zucchini have completely cooled before adding the dressing. Then, snuggle a single layer of zucchini strips next to each other on your serving dish. Drizzle a small amount of the dressing over them. You do not have to use all of the dressing—just about a teaspoon for each slice. Repeat the process by stacking another layer of zucchini on top of the first one. When you've stacked and drizzled all the strips, you're ready to serve them to your guests.

Unless you've made so many strips that your leftovers last more than two days, do not put them in the refrigerator; leave them at room temperature. A cold environment makes the zucchini go limp, so my advice is to make full use of your long vegetable strips while they're still firm and crunchy.

Store the leftover dressing for up to three days at room temperature. Beyond that, keep it in the refrigerator. Use it for various grilled dishes, such as lamb and seafood. Make sure to mix the dressing well before you add it to any prepared dishes.

When you try this recipe, I guarantee you'll fall in love with it, as I did. Especially if you remember my story of the two young boys with large bulges in their pants, or the times I peered over a wise woman's shoulder to learn her zucchini secrets.

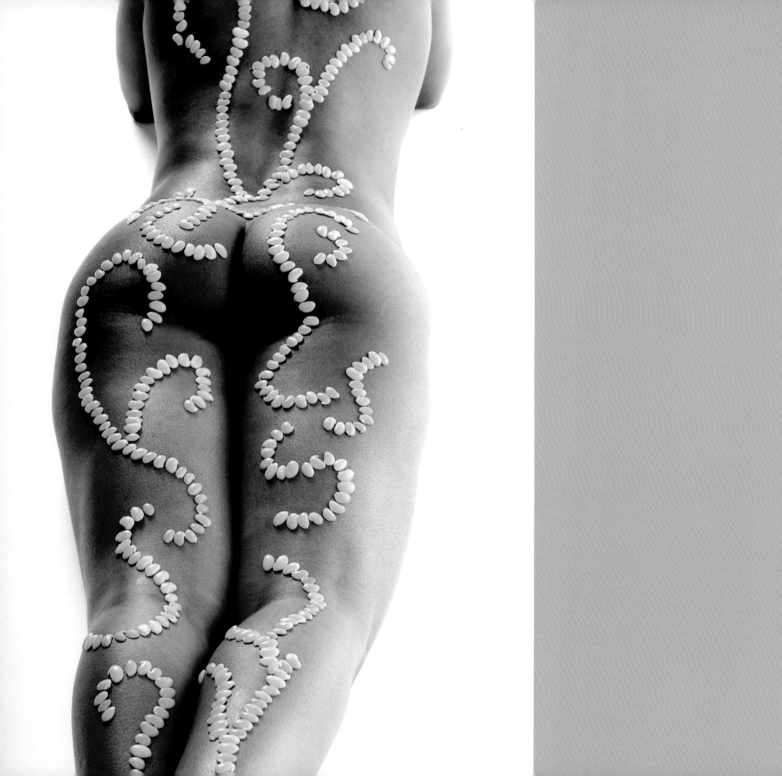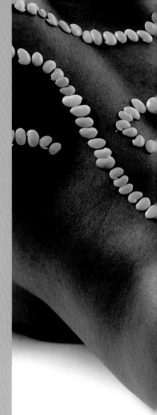

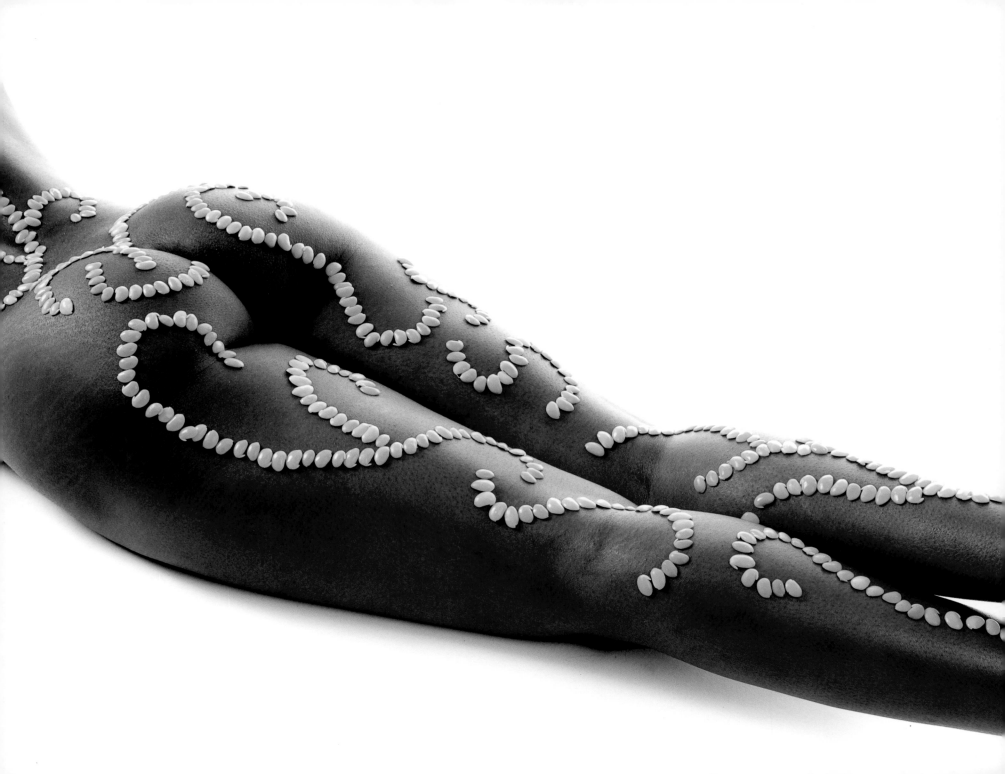

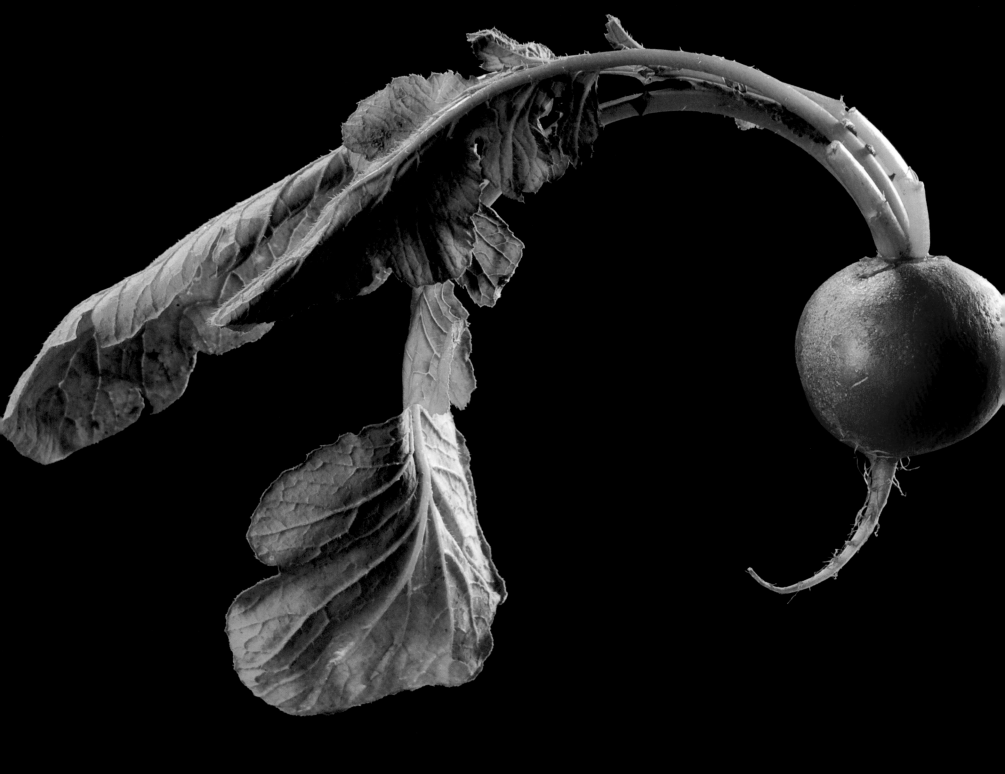

RADISHES

Radishes, women, and really salty potato chips are addicting. I indulge myself in the first two but seldom in the third. I didn't always hold the radish in such high regard, however. The relationship developed slowly, but deeply, and now this zesty little vegetable is dear to my heart.

There's a radish for everyone, I believe, if you keep your mind open and experiment with the abundance of varieties: round, skinny, long, or pear-shaped; yellow, white, red, or pink; crunchy or soft; sharp, mild, or somewhere in between.

To bring color to your kitchen and a smile to your face, place several types of fresh radishes in a bowl on your table or counter. They'll look beautiful as they snuggle together, just like a pile of people snuggling during an evening of love.

LEMON RADISHES

USE A SHARP KNIFE to slice about 10 radishes very finely. Place them in a bowl and add enough olive oil to coat them. Add 1 to 2 cloves of smashed garlic and plenty of sea salt, followed by 1 tablespoon of fresh lemon. Fold everything together, cover the bowl, and let it sit at room temperature for at least two hours or even as long as three days.

You will notice the radishes are covered with juice—this is great. It means the salt was doing its job to release the juice from the radishes. Sip some of this juice to see if you can taste the salt and the garlic. Add more if you think it needs it, but don't go overboard adding more garlic unless that is what you prefer. Note that, once it is marinating, the flavor will get stronger every day.

This dish is perfect to add to bread or grilled seafood, or to simply eat as a side dish. If so, you might choose to add extra olive oil. You can never go wrong with good Italian olive oil.

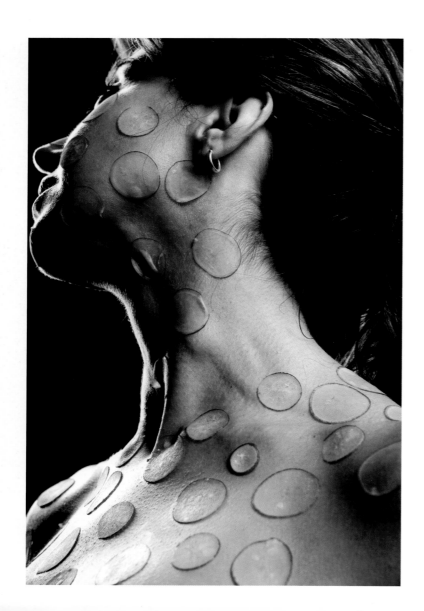
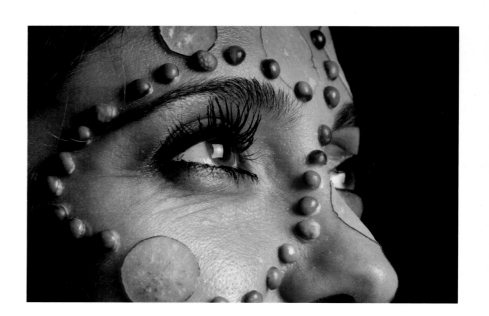

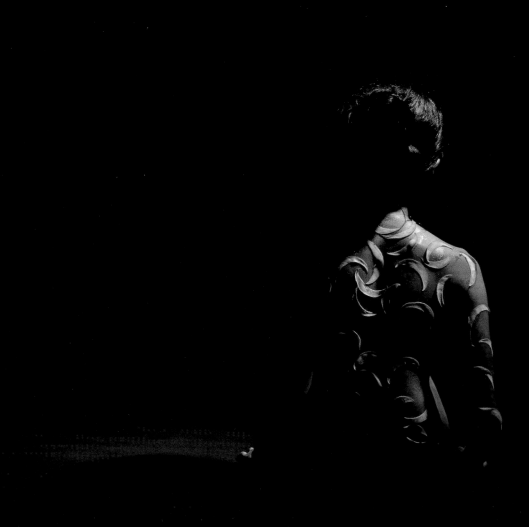

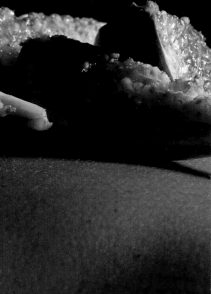

They shall sit every man under his vine and under his fig tree.
—The Bible, Micah 4:4

The fig is a very secretive fruit. As you see it standing growing, you feel at once it is symbolic: And it seems male. But when you come to know it better, you agree with the Romans, it is female. —D. H. Lawrence

I TRULY ADORE THIS FRUIT. In fact, I chose *La Figa* as the name for my catering business and then this book because it brings to mind images both of this exquisite fruit and of a beautiful woman—sometimes together, in the same image.

Where I come from in Italy, fig trees are everywhere. They come in a wonderful variety of luscious colors: red, purple, yellow, green, almost white, and almost black. In Southern Italy alone, there are at least a hundred different types of figs.

Some are small and super sweet with a honey flavor so intense that, once you bite into it, you must pause for a few seconds—the pleasure is overwhelming. The flesh is thin and packed with vitamins so these figs are usually eaten with the skin on. The bigger ones are sweet as well but not as intense; their flavors are fresh and pungent, and the texture is grainier. Then there are the Colombo figs, which are the giant ones, like the size of a pear. It is best to eat these with the skin off because their flesh is very thick.

I most certainly have a sweet spot for this tasty fruit. Delicious, sexy, versatile, intriguing: figs have it all. They are happy in the company of honey, sugar, thin proscuitto, and sweet spices (such as ginger, cinnamon, and cloves), as well as with the sharpness of citrus fruits. In my mind, fresh figs eaten with prosciutto di Parma are the most perfect and sensual combination. I also like to grill figs dipped in a balsamic reduction with panettone.

A fig cannot ripen once it is picked from its tree so select already ripened ones from the market. The best fruit will feel soft, like baby cheeks.

If you're lucky, you won't have to worry about choosing the right one at the market; you will find the perfect fig dangling from a branch, yet to be picked. When I go home to Neviano in the summertime, I love to eat figs right from the tree, reaching up with my mouth and not using my hands. My lips envelop the delicious drop of honey inevitably hanging from the bottom of the fig. I try to leave the skin intact as I slowly suck that sweet nectar. Mmm…I can taste it right now.

There are many ways to eat a fig, but I recommend one of the most popular: simply grab the neck and pull to split the fruit in half. Enjoy the bright color of the glistening flesh and then scrape it into your mouth, leaving the skin behind. Savor the unique texture and intense flavor on your tongue for a few seconds and then slowly let it slide down your throat.

In Italy, the fig is not only celebrated because it is a delicious fruit, but because it is reminiscent of a woman's genitalia. This is a compliment because it suggests that a woman is very beautiful. *Che bella figa che è* means "what a beautiful woman she is." In Italian, *la figa* intimates something fresh and beautiful, as in the whole body of a lovely woman. Likewise, *che bel fico che è* means what a beautiful man he is; *fico* is the fig tree itself—strong and thrusting.

Figs are one of those glorious foods that I could eat every day, just like I could eat a woman, and there's no better way to eat a fig than directly from a beautiful woman's body. I love it when both meanings of fig come together.

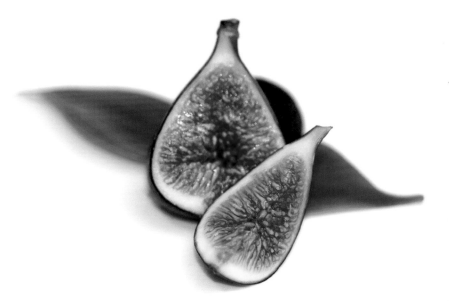

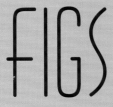

FIGS

FROM THEIR SHAPE AND TEXTURE to their taste and fragrance, figs are a sensual fruit in every way imaginable. One of my favorite ways to eat them is right off the tree, but other methods are tasty too, especially if they involve a woman.

Figs are versatile, however, so be sure to try them in combination with other flavors. I believe they are one of the best-kept secrets in America…and I love to explore a good secret and discover its hidden treasures.

If you ever find yourself with more figs than you can eat, use them to make fig jam. For the tastiest jam, be sure to choose only figs that are soft, ripe, and sweet. Or use your figs to make Drunken Figs, a perfect companion for all types of meat or desserts.

FIG JAM

IN A LARGE SAUCEPAN, combine 2 lbs. of peeled figs, 1 lb. of sugar, the juice of 1 or 2 large lemons (depending on your preference), 2 teaspoons of cinnamon, and 1 bay leaf.

Bring to a boil and then simmer slowly for about 15 minutes. Stir gently. The jam should be chunky.

Cool completely and spoon the jam into sterilized jars. Store the jars in the refrigerator. The jam will last up to 6 weeks.

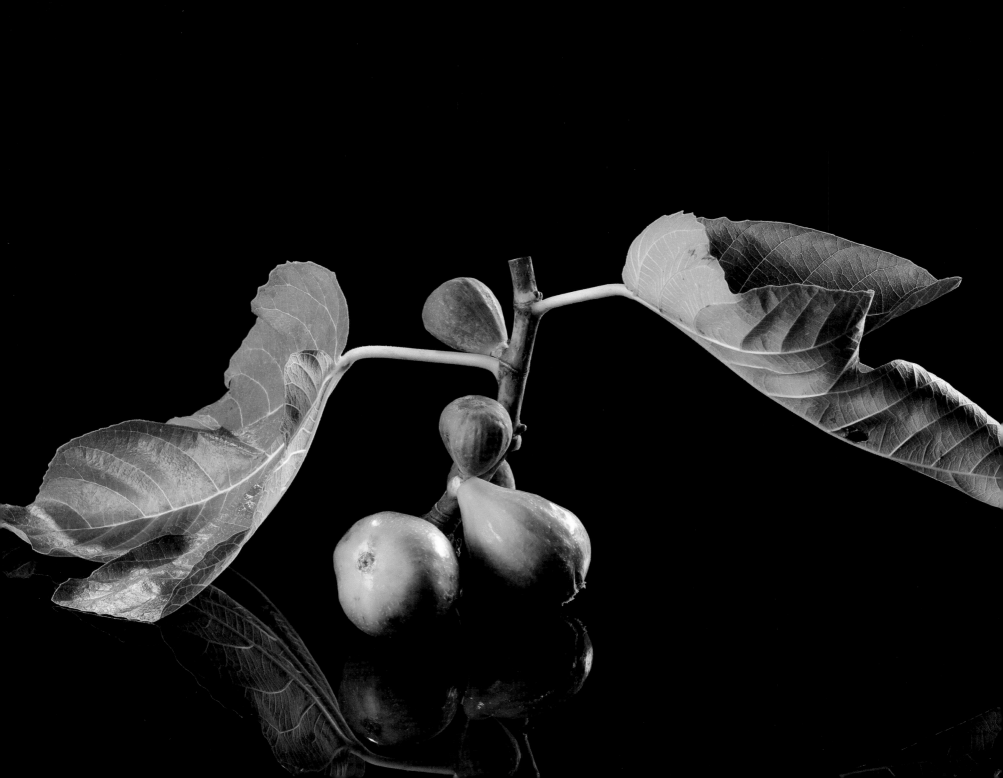

DRUNKEN FIGS

Place 2 lbs. of dry, black mission figs in a glass jar.

In a medium saucepan, combine 3 quarts of inexpensive port wine, 1 to 2 cups of honey, 3 cinnamon sticks, 7 to 10 cloves, 5 whole star anise, and 1/2 of the skin of both a small orange and a large lemon. Bring the mixture to a boil and then simmer until the amount is reduced by half. Cool to room temperature. Poor the liquid into the fig jars and cover them tightly. Keep them closed for at least two days.

The drunken figs are now quite drunk and ready to be used in many seductive and sensual ways. You will have plenty of opportunities to share them with friends, since the figs will last all year in the jar at room temperature if they remain covered by the drunken juice.

A little hint: they go well with duck confit, gorgonzola, mushrooms, steak, and human lips.

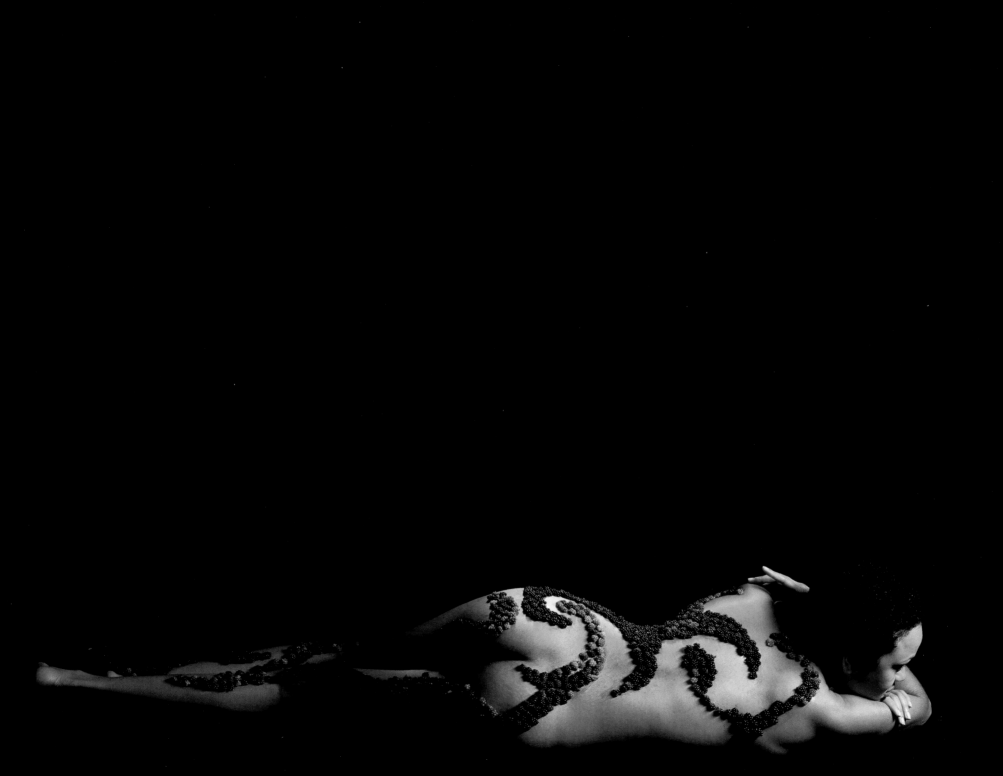

ARE FOOD AND SEX equally important to you?

I often ask this question and many people say yes. "Food and sex are all I think about when I wake up in the morning," said a lovely woman I met in Mexico. Another friend said, "Oh, yeah, they're all I want."

Most people immediately note that food and sex can be very pleasurable, and it's true. Our need for food and sex goes way beyond pleasure: we wouldn't exist without them. They are essential for our survival.

Growing up on the land, however, taught me that surviving isn't enough. We must also thrive, just like the plants and trees my family and I cultivated on parcels of farmland in Italy. To thrive as people, we need *healthy* food and *healthy* sex.

Let's face it, there is plenty of bad food and plenty of bad sex. Just because we're eating and procreating and surviving doesn't mean we're healthy. We have all made poor food choices at one time or another—and we have also probably made some bad decisions when it comes to being intimate with someone we should have taken a pass on.

Eating unhealthy food might make us feel good at the moment, but, afterwards, our bodies feel miserable and we function poorly, sometimes without realizing it.

The same thing is true for sex. It is important to be careful about who you choose to share your bed with: if the match isn't right, it might feel good for a moment but then you'll pay for it afterwards. Just like the body can have an allergic reaction to food, I believe we can have an allergic reaction to sex with the wrong person. Some people simply have a toxic energy, so it's best to avoid them. They are truly harmful to your health.

Nutrition affects not only our bodies but love and lovemaking, too. When we eat healthily, we feel good because our bodies are happy with the nutrition we've provided. We have more energy to play, and our sexual appetite immediately improves. When we have nutritious food in our bodies and we make love with others who are good for us, we have brought together the *healthy ingredients for gourmet sex*, as I like to call it.

Try adding more of these fruits and vegetables—garlic, grapes, beets, berries, artichokes, tomatoes, red peppers, broccoli, and spinach—to your diet. Other great choices include seafood, especially salmon and herring. Dark chocolate is excellent, but in moderation, of course. I've heard of studies showing that women who eat a small amount of chocolate each day report significantly more sexual desire and better overall sexual function than women who don't.

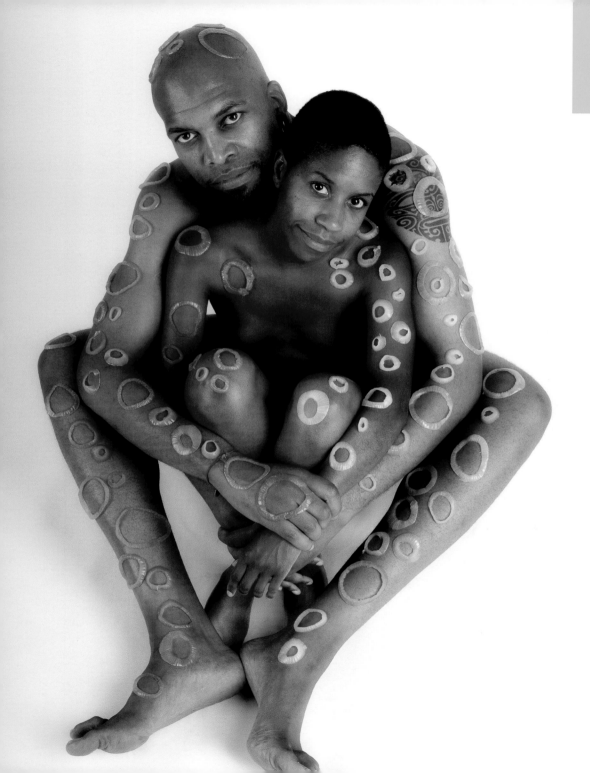

Chocolate is also a natural antidepressant. I include all of these food choices in my diet on a regular basis.

Libido-inhibiting food, such as sugar, may taste wonderful, but it's not so good for the bedroom. Other things to avoid include salt, saturated fat, highly processed food, heavy cream sauces, and fatty meats, like bacon. I suggest having these in moderation—just enough to satisfy an occasional craving.

Another similarity between sex and food is that we have mistakenly been trained to think youth and beauty are more desirable. Someone who is older, less handsome, or imperfect has less value. But the opposite is often true. I know a lot of people who, by society's standards, are not the most desirable, but they are very real, very attractive, and very tasty.

The same is true with food. A hothouse tomato you find at a grocery store looks terrific—so pretty, so plump, so ripe and juicy. Guess what? It has no flavor! There is no comparison between this tasteless tomato and the less-than-perfect version grown on an organic farm or by a local farmer.

When you share your body with a lover, you are also sharing your own body's nutrition and health, whether it's good or bad. When you prepare food for a lover, the nutritional value of this food will be reflected in your lover's libido and, thus, in the sex the two of you have.

Food is love. Love is sex. Sex is food. They are all linked. And we are all of them.

The truth is not so much that there are similarities between food and sex; it is that they are one and the same.

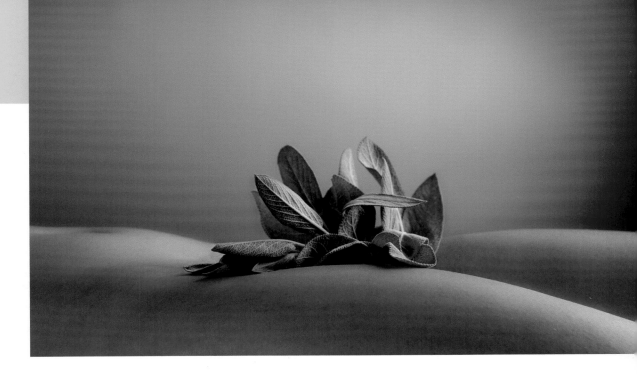

I KNOW A LOT OF PEOPLE WHO, BY SOCIETY'S STANDARDS, ARE NOT THE MOST DESIRABLE, BUT THEY ARE VERY REAL, VERY ATTRACTIVE, AND VERY TASTY.

So I encourage you to take pleasure in healthy food and healthy sex. They are essential to your well-being, and to that of your lover or lovers too.

Here is a recipe for spending a day with a special person—someone who is tasty and attractive to you and who appreciates this symbiotic relationship between food and sex. These are examples of my *healthy ingredients for gourmet sex*:

10:00 a.m. Walk or run three to six miles, or whatever distance is comfortable for both of you.

11:00 a.m. Shower. Together, if you prefer.

11:30 a.m. Make lunch: a green salad with non-creamy dressing; simple brown rice with a fresh vegetable; red or yellow lentils with fresh Italian parsley and good olive oil; a fruit platter with honey.

12:30 p.m. Eat lunch. Feed each other.

1:30 p.m. Retreat to the bedroom, where you have put fresh, white sheets on the bed.

Later…naptime. Hold each other and spoon.

Take care of yourselves and each other. Good food and good sex are essential, intertwined, and the difference between surviving and thriving.

I give you permission to eat and permission to make love.

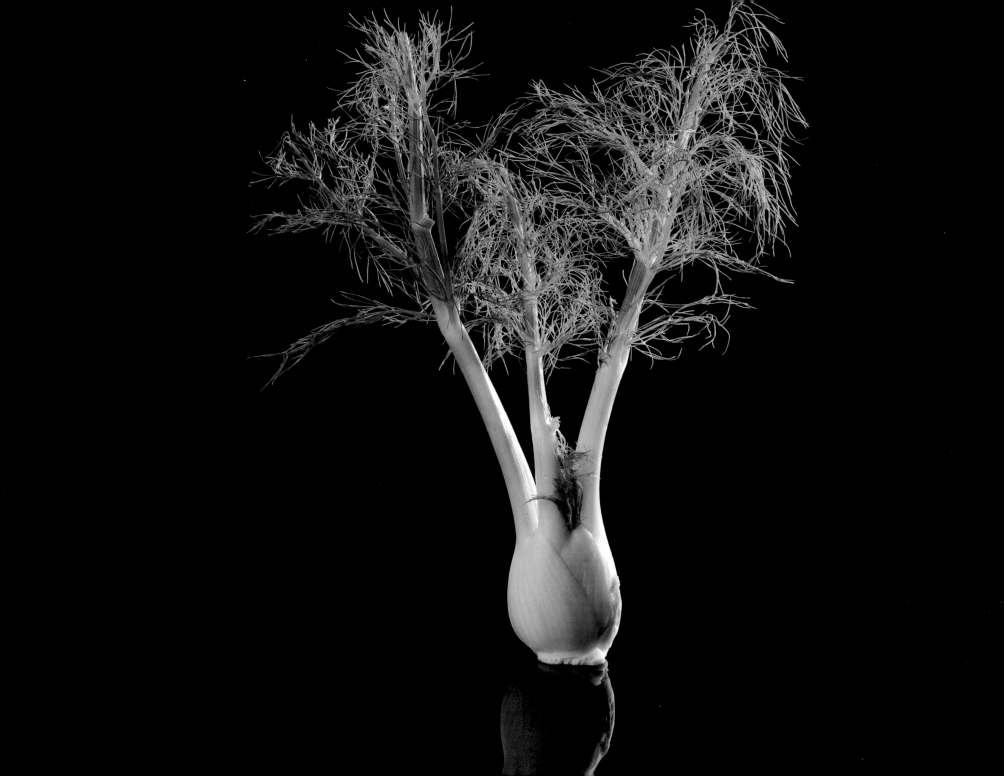

FENNEL

LIKE A THOUGHTFUL LOVER, fennel meets many needs. It's a spice, an herb, and a vegetable, all in one plant. Sometimes it tastes like aniseed and licorice, only more delicate. Many people know and love the airy green leaves that are used to flavor recipes, but I've found fewer people who are aware of the tasty uses of the white plant bulb itself.

In the wintertime, when fennel—or *finocchio*, in Italian—was abundant, my mother incorporated different sections of the plant into wonderful recipes on an almost daily basis. She added it to meat stew, seafood cioppino, or boiled rapini, for example, as a way to give a little perfume to the dish.

We also ate the raw bulb of the finocchio plant with our hands—like an apple—at the end of the meal. I still enjoy breaking off a finger-size chunk of the plant's core and eating it by itself or with a crunchy baguette. I could eat raw fennel in one form or another every day.

FENNEL SALAD

My mother often made this quick and easy recipe. Today, I use it when I'm short on time or when company arrives unexpectedly—or when I want a flavorful reminder of those earthy and bountiful winter days in Southern Italy.

After thinly slicing the inner layers of the fennel bulb, mix them with butter lettuce, then toss with very good olive oil, sea salt, and a few drops of lemon juice.

The freshness of this simple salad appeals to my palate and leaves an aromatic taste in my mouth for several hours—a fresh flavor I can enjoy and share with the person I'm kissing.

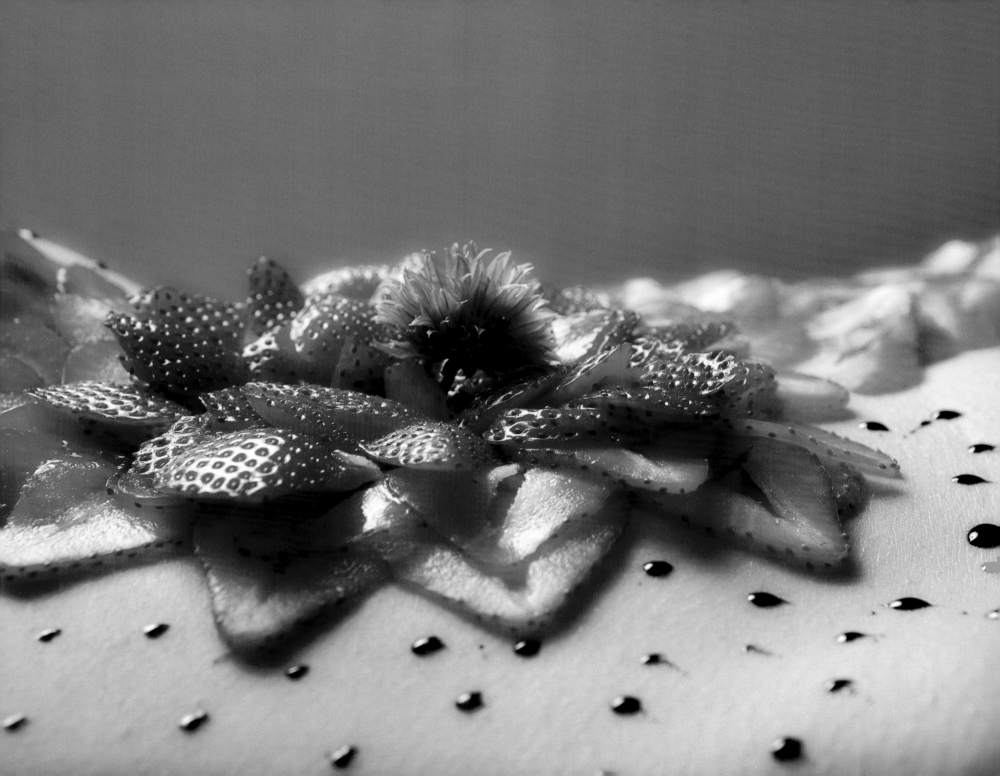

Doubtless God could have made a better berry…but doubtless God never did.
—William Allen Butler

AHH…THE MAGIC OF THE STRAWBERRY

The strawberry has long been one of the world's most widely known and respected berries, and rightly so. Eating these delightful little bundles of flavor certainly tops my list of uses, but humans have also discovered a multitude of ways to achieve health, happiness, and pleasure from the strawberry.

Tradition has it that Madame Tallien, a prominent social figure during the rule of the French Emperor Napoleon, regularly bathed in fresh strawberry juice, using up to twenty-two pounds per basin.

Entire societies have touted the medicinal value of the wild strawberry and its leaves and roots. The ancient Romans, in particular, relied on berries to relieve the symptoms of depression, dizziness, fevers, infections, kidney stones, gout, and liver disease. My ancestors were a wise people.

Did you know the strawberry is actually a member of the rose family? Or that the strawberry is the only fruit with its seeds—all two hundred of them, on average—on the outside? …Mamma mia! So much power in a little package.

Rumor has it that if you break a double strawberry in half and share it with a member of the opposite sex, you will fall in love with each other. I tried that once with someone I was attracted to when I worked as a chef at a large, corporate hotel in Seattle. Instead of ending up in each other's arms, I ended up on the verge of a sexual harassment charge. I chuckle about it today, but it was not funny then. My advice? Make sure you know this person well enough, and you approach him or her outside of the corporate workplace. When you are successful, invite me to your wedding, or at least to your home for a party. I will bring strawberries.

FINDING YOUR PERFECT STRAWBERRY

The most fragrant and flavorful strawberries are those you pick yourself or purchase at your local strawberry field or farmer's market. Truly farm-fresh strawberries are only hours old, with little or no handling or traveling, and you will taste, see, and smell the difference.

Look for plump, bright red, and fully ripe berries. The caps should be green, still attached, and fresh-looking. The size of the strawberry is not important because all strawberries, both large and small, can be sweet and juicy. I prefer small, dark ones because I know they are going to be awesome.

If you buy strawberries in the store, make sure they are super fresh. Organic *and* super fresh is an even better combination. A good strawberry that's ready to eat will be a bright, darkish red color, and firm. If the strawberry is soft, it is too ripe. You might get lucky and it will taste great, but more than likely it won't. Or it will go bad in no time.

When you buy a pint, make sure there is not a single rotten berry in the bunch because the others will quickly follow its lead. To make my selection, I empty the entire pint to confirm there aren't any bruised or rotten ones, and then I simply refill the container. A quicker method is to see if the bottom of the carton is wet. A soggy bottom is a sure sign these strawberries will not meet your needs or bring you the pleasure you deserve.

My Strawberry Art with a Lovely Friend

The strawberry is one of the first ingredients Matt and I used in a photo shoot. Back then, we asked each model which edible ingredient she or he would be in a future life and then used that food item in the photo shoot.

"The strawberry!" our sexy, amazing model replied. This was before we had a photography studio, so we did this shoot on my kitchen table. It was quite a challenge, especially for the model, because she had to remain perfectly still while I applied the strawberries.

Sliced strawberries are very slick and slippery, so getting them to stick to her beautiful skin was a test of everyone's patience. Then and now, I use only edible ingredients to adhere the food to each model's body, and the sugar water concoction I was using that day did not do the trick.

I suddenly remembered a recipe I'd recently developed to use with strawberries: a balsamic vinegar reduction. We tried it and…presto!

The combination was perfect and the results were fantastic. So wonderful, in fact, we decided to incorporate dots of the reduction itself into the body art, in addition to using it to adhere the strawberries to our adventurous model. I called her my ladybug.

Then I had this crazy idea to carry our model into my backyard—to an outdoor setting worthy of our ladybug. Matt and I lifted her, placed in a red tub that appears in a photo on page 169, and carried her down the stairs. The woman wasn't heavy, but the tub was. Despite the risk of injury to herself, she was a great sport, and we laughed a lot as we struggled to avoid squishing her strawberries or smearing her ladybug dots.

In the end, neither bodies nor fruit were hurt, and the results of that day's photo shoot, which you can see on the opposite page, were fantastic. In fact, the positive feedback we got on these early photos was one of the reasons we decided to turn our little photo project into a full-sized book.

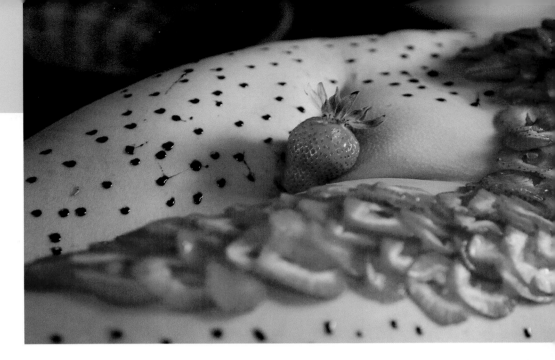
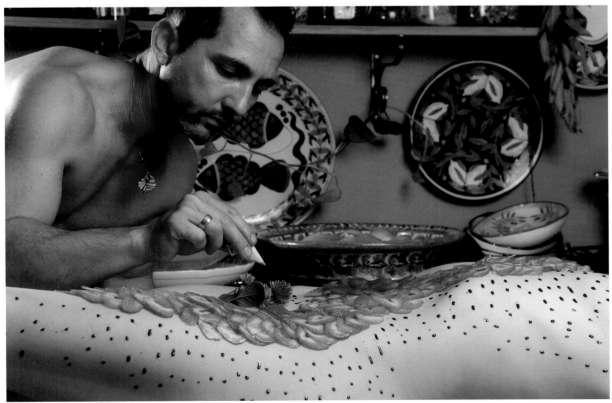

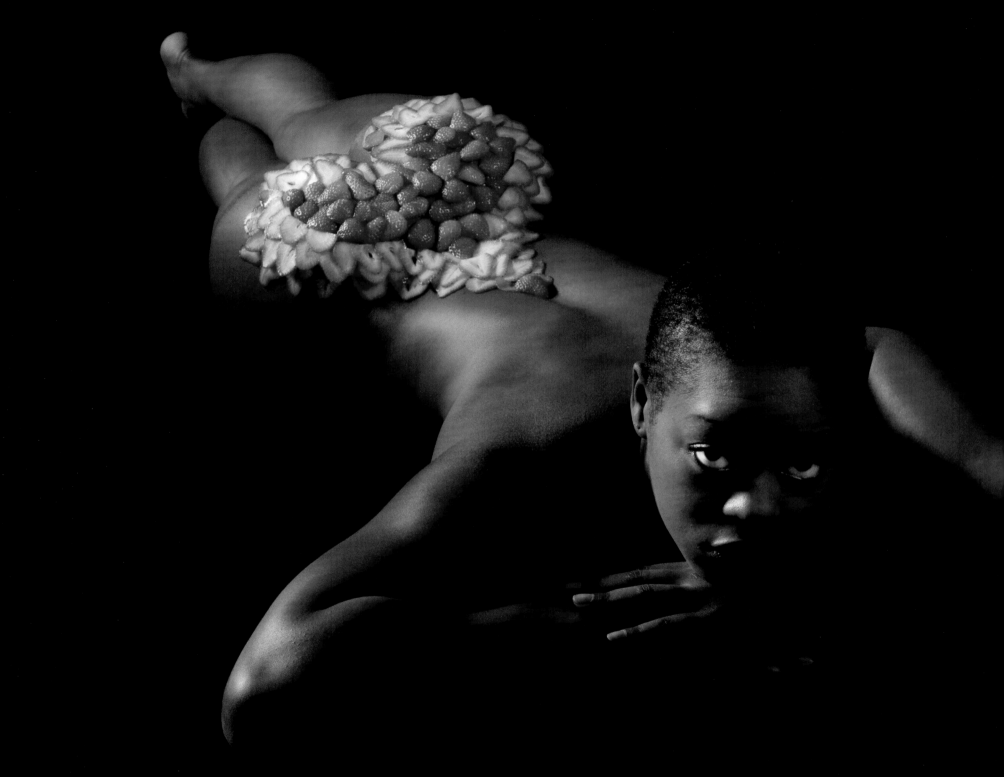

STRAWBERRIES

THERE IS NO COMPARISON between a perfect strawberry and one that is combined with other ingredients—the sweetness and smell of that single work of art is all we really need to fully appreciate this vibrant berry. Try this and see if you agree: The next time you come across a fragrant and richly colored specimen, wash it in cold water. As you eat it, close your eyes and breathe gently through your nose so you can savor the taste and the fragrance at the same time. Heaven on earth, right?

On the other hand, too much of any one thing does not leave room for opportunity or inspiration, so we often seek both by combining a special food item with other ingredients. If we're lucky, serendipity occurs and all five of our senses rejoice.

One of the most memorable recipes I developed during my career while working as a pastry chef at the Four Seasons Olympic Hotel in Seattle features strawberries with a balsamic vinegar reduction…although giving birth to this simple blend of flavors was not without labor pains.

In those days, I had a lot of room to be creative— if I was willing to come in early or stay late. The daily routine and pressure of creating, preparing, and presenting innovative desserts for two of that elegant hotel's fine-dining restaurants meant recipe development was often done on my own time.

The executive chef of the hotel had great connections with an organic farm, which brought us exquisite produce. In this instance, it was strawberries.

Oh, my God, they were tiny and dark red—one bite was like a sweet, wet, yummy kiss. I wanted to retain these strawberries' own precious flavor and serve them in as natural a state as possible, which meant using very few ingredients in the dessert.

The first attempt did not work: a wine reduction with honey was too sweet. A bottle of balsamic vinegar caught my eye, so I used it instead of the wine and with only half the honey.

The result was surprising—a wonderful balance of sweetness and acidity. But something was missing, some sort of spice. Nothing in the pastry shop produced anything that met my expectations, however.

Fuck it, I thought. *I'm going to add some freshly cracked black pepper as a last ridiculous try.*

Guess what? It was perfect!

The pepper, as it turned out, was like a benediction I sprinkled on top, just before serving the unusual combination of strawberries and good balsamic vinegar.

I've used this recipe often, but only when I have excellent strawberries.

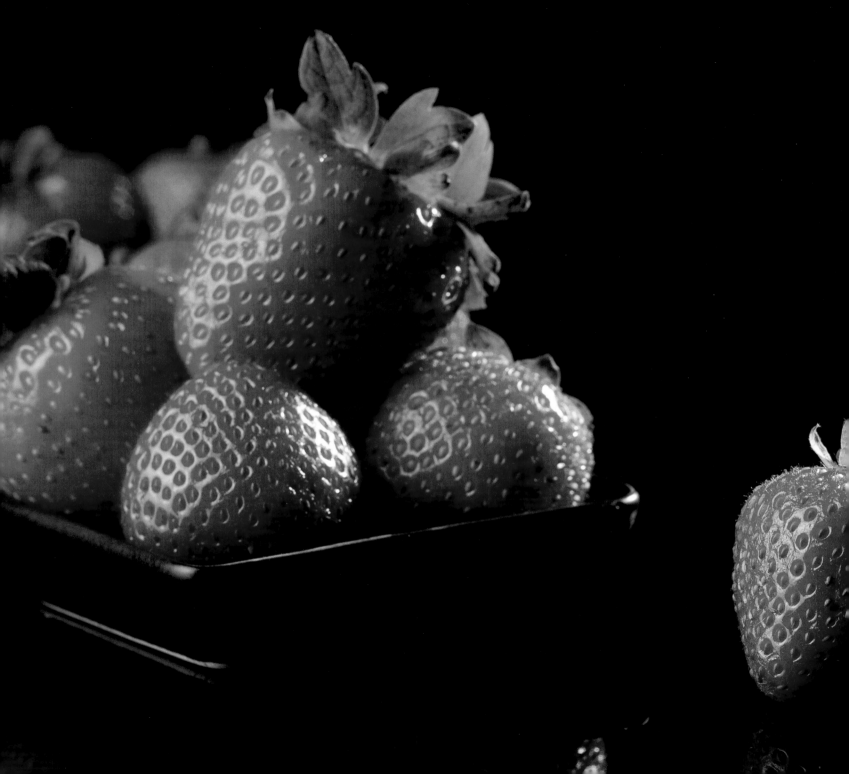

STRAWBERRIES WITH A BALSAMIC VINEGAR REDUCTION

{

IN A SMALL OR MEDIUM POT, combine 2 cups of decent or good quality balsamic vinegar—I prefer that from Modena, Italy—with 3/4 cup of honey. Reduce the mixture down to 3/4 cup. Let it cool completely.

Slice a pint of tiny, dark red strawberries, if they're available, and arrange them on individual dessert dishes for your guests.

Drizzle the reduction over the sliced strawberries, but be careful—the reduction has a lot of flavor, so a little goes a long way. Add a small amount of freshly ground pepper to the top. Serve it alone or with very good quality vanilla ice cream.

I predict the shiny, dark syrup and rich, red berries will beckon your guests, who will already be smiling in pleasurable anticipation.

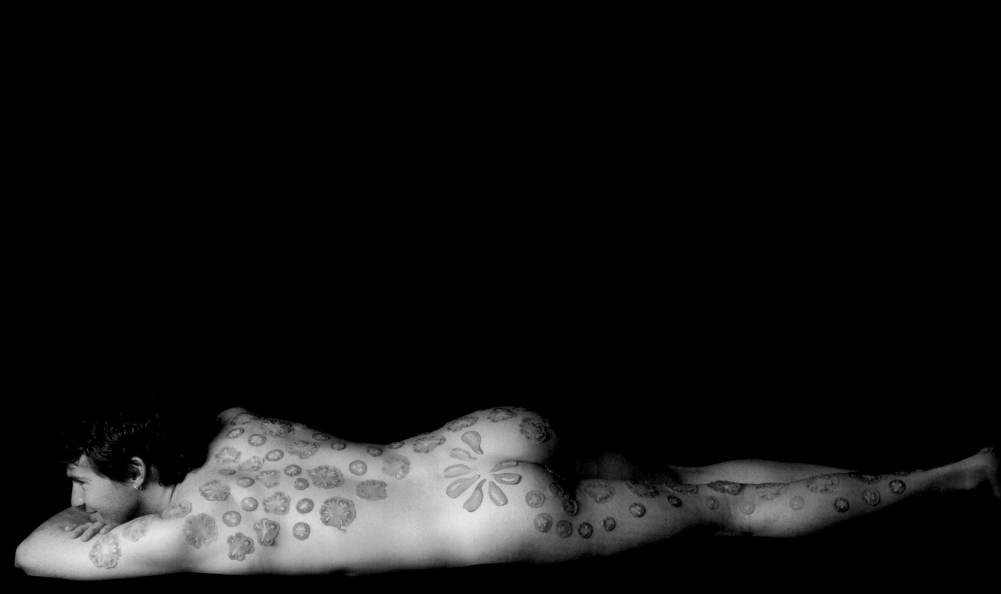

TOMATOES EXCITE ME. When I hold a plump, ripe tomato in my hand and take a bite of it—whoa!—I am astounded at the rush of flavor, the gush of juice.

After that first surge of pleasure, I am transported to my childhood in Italy, where tomatoes were a staple we ate in one form or another nearly every day. The tangy smell of a deep red tomato freshly plucked from the vine, the feel of the sun's warming rays on the juicy ball in my hand, and the crunchy sound as my teeth break through the thin yet durable skin… ahh. Unforgettable.

America—the land of plenty—has plenty of perfectly formed and temptingly colored, flavorless tomatoes that barely resemble the tomatoes of Italy (or other places around the world that value taste over looks). Even during the summer, when American tomatoes are in season and can potentially stand up to their European cousins, they fall flat. These weak tomatoes are grown in hothouses—sometimes in North America, sometimes overseas—picked too early, and left to ripen in warehouses, far from the sun, dirt, and rain. They are too removed from the earth, and they've certainly lost whatever taste and fragrance they once had. Don't be fooled by these year-round tomatoes; they're an attractive shade of red, uniformly colored and sized, perfectly formed…and perfectly terrible to eat.

Now that you know how I really feel about the out-of-season tomatoes that are typically sold in most grocery stores, I can assure you there are other alternatives that are practically right in your own backyard. (In fact, many Americans—even those in urban areas—choose to grace their backyards, patios, and their meals with fragrant, *real* tomatoes they've grown themselves.) Your local farmer's market is another great choice, since that produce has typically been picked within the past few hours and may very well have been grown organically. Some smaller, gourmet-style grocery stores often buy from local farmers, so that might be another option for you.

I urge you to make the extra effort to find real tomatoes, full of the flavor of the earth and with tasty imperfections you won't see on those other tomatoes. You will thank me for it when you lose your virginity to a real tomato! You'll tell me you never knew it could be this good…and I will remember my own tomato experiences growing up on a farm.

Like everyone in our small, southern town, my father grew many types of tomatoes. For most Italians, the tomato is one of the main fruit ingredients in our daily lives, especially the San Marzano tomato, which works best for sauces. My mother used this variety of tomato in the sauce she ladled over *spaghetti al dente*—such a warm, juicy pleasure in our mouths. Years later, I finally figured out how—and why—we regularly ate giant servings of pasta at lunchtime: the sweet, delicate tomato sauce, with its fresh basil perfume and scent of olive oil, lured us into heaping more and more pasta on our plates so we would have an excuse to request more sauce. We also competed to see who could do the best job scraping his plate clean by using a chunk of bread to soak up the extra sauce. Even now, the aroma lingers in my memory, and I hunger for my mother's tomato sauce.

Once or twice a year, every family in Southern Italy, it seemed, made its own supply of tomato sauce, hoping the fruits of the day's labor would last until the next year. Even though the day was quite hectic and very long, we had a lot of fun. Everyone in the family worked because there were so many jobs to do, and we often switched back and forth, taking turns, so we could do a little bit of everything. It was never boring.

Starting early in the day, we washed every tomato, then held it under water and squished it to remove the seeds—a process called *sbinchulare*. Another person was in charge of stirring the tomatoes cooking in a giant pot, and someone else washed and dried the dusty bottles from the previous year. After that, another person—often a child—added one leaf of basil to each clean bottle. By now, an adult was passing the cooked tomatoes into the smashing machine to separate the

skin from the pulp. Someone else filled each bottle with the aromatic sauce. Another person sealed the bottle and tapped the lid to make sure the seal was good.

We usually filled about 250 one-liter bottles, which meant we could have a tomato-based food item 250 days a year. I did not like to think about the other 115 days that would lack this cheery, red sauce.

Of all the sauces my mother makes, my favorite is her tomato sauce with sweet onion and *ricotta sciante*, or fermented ricotta, which is a specialty in Southern Italy. The fermented ricotta is so powerful that only one teaspoon is needed in a batch of sauce that will serve five people. It is incredibly good, and many people—including me—find it addictive. Whenever I go home to Neviano, my mother makes *spaghetti alla ricotta sciante* with this sauce and tops it with pecorino cheese. I have to say, it is orgasmic—it really is! As soon as I take my first bite, it's as if I've never eaten it before and will never have it again, so I must shovel it in quickly. Then I get a hold of myself and slow down because I want to taste everything and make it last as long as it can—just like sweet, yummy sex. Trust me, if you ever have a chance to taste this sauce, you will understand.

As a child, I thought my life was hard, but I now see how fortunate I was to be part of the process of bringing *real* tomatoes to my family's table.

Tomato, I love you as much as I love a lover. And that is a lot.

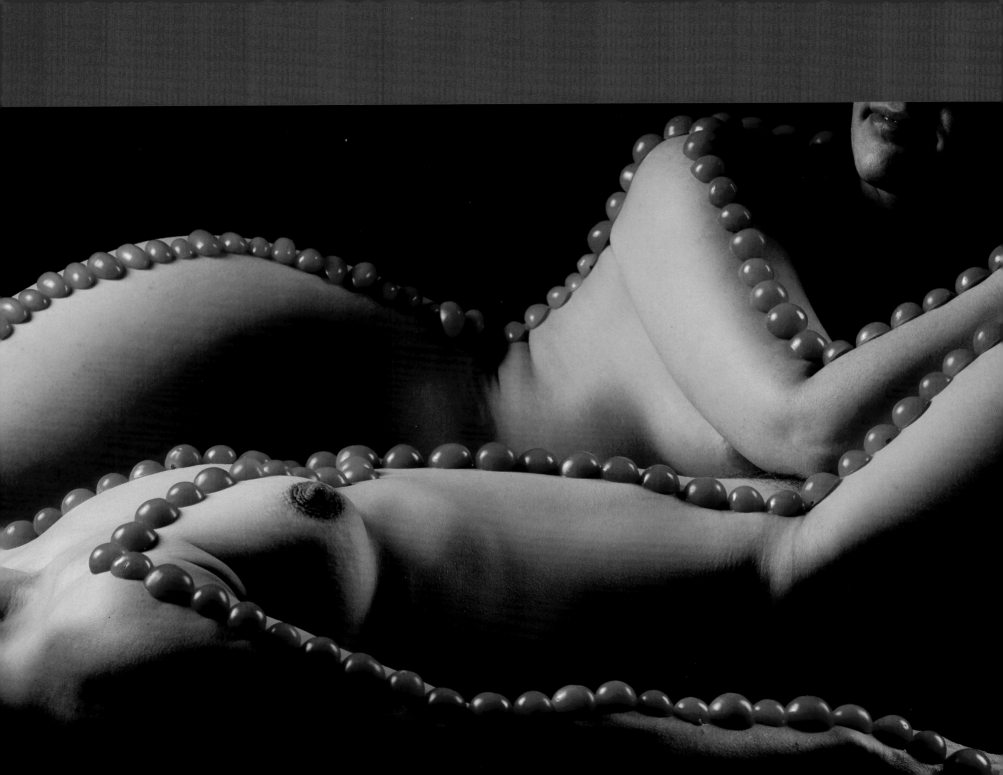

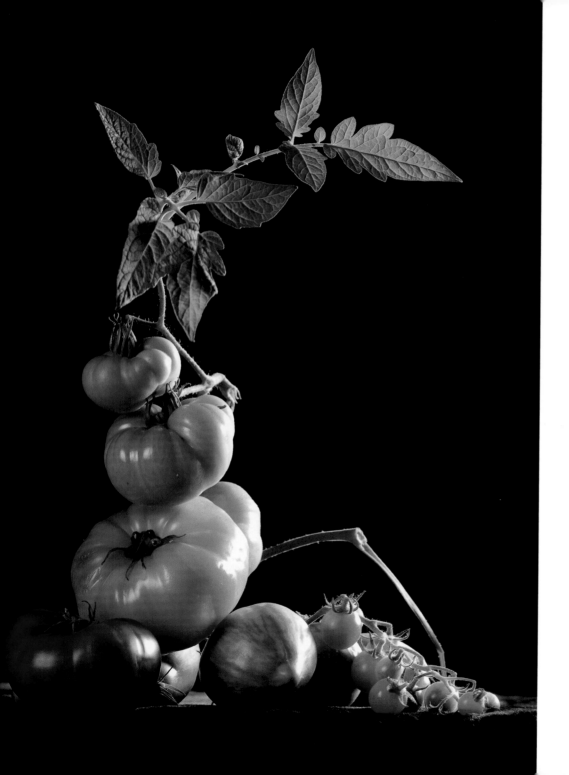

IF SOMEONE WERE TO ASK ME what I would like to eat at my last meal, I would immediately answer: The All-Tomato Salad. If that person asked me why, I would explain it's because the freshness of the ingredients remind me of my childhood on the farm. The All-Tomato Salad also embodies the wonderful talent my mother has for creating magic from basic, farm-fresh ingredients. Beyond everything else, The All-Tomato Salad is an homage to my mother for her love, guidance, and nurturing.

With this recipe, the more types of tomatoes you use, the more complex the flavor—just like with people. Each one contributes something to the whole, which creates more diverse and satisfying results.

When you're at the market to choose your tomatoes, put one up to your nose and mouth, and breathe in. If you don't smell anything, that tomato will taste bland and fleshy—flavorless, basically. Refrigeration reduces a tomato's natural flavors and the only way to improve the situation is to add a lot of extra salt, which will overpower every other taste and isn't healthy for us anyway.

If the tomato *smells* like a tomato, however, and there aren't any bruises or obvious problems, you probably have a good one in your hand. Go for it. This is assuming tomatoes are in season; if not, you need to be very selective.

Before you start making your All-Tomato Salad, sample one of your purchases. Salt a piece of bread, add a little olive oil and the slices of one of your tomatoes. The taste will send you soaring above the clouds and flying to heaven.

Remember, never refrigerate the tomato.

TOMATOES

THE ALL-TOMATO SALAD

{

THIS RECIPE IS VERY SIMPLE, especially once you know the secret: use Heirloom tomatoes, preferably those grown organically. If you can't find Heirlooms, use several different varieties of organic tomatoes.

To serve 4 people, you'll need 1 lb. of fresh tomatoes. Slice the big ones about 1/2-inch thick, cut the smaller ones in half, and leave the smallest ones whole. Slice 2 stalks of celery about 1/3-inch thick, and thinly slice half of a medium-size red onion; add the celery and onions to the pile of tomatoes slices.

Put these ingredients in your favorite bowl and then add 1 to 2 tablespoons of dry oregano, 1/4 cup of very good quality extra virgin olive oil, 1 teaspoon of chili flakes (or more, if you wish), and about 8 to 10 leaves of fresh basil, broken in medium-size pieces with your hands. Add sea salt to taste.

With clean hands, gently fold the salad. If you want to know if the salad is perfectly seasoned, have another person lick your messy fingers and give you his or her opinion. I lick my own finger, too, because it tastes so good and so we can compare notes to determine if the salad has the right amount of salt, chili, and oregano.

Let it sit for at least 30 minutes before serving and sharing. If you can't wait that long, dip a chunk of crusty bread into the juice after about 20 minutes, close your eyes, and enjoy.

I could eat this salad until my belly explodes, and sometimes I've just about done that.

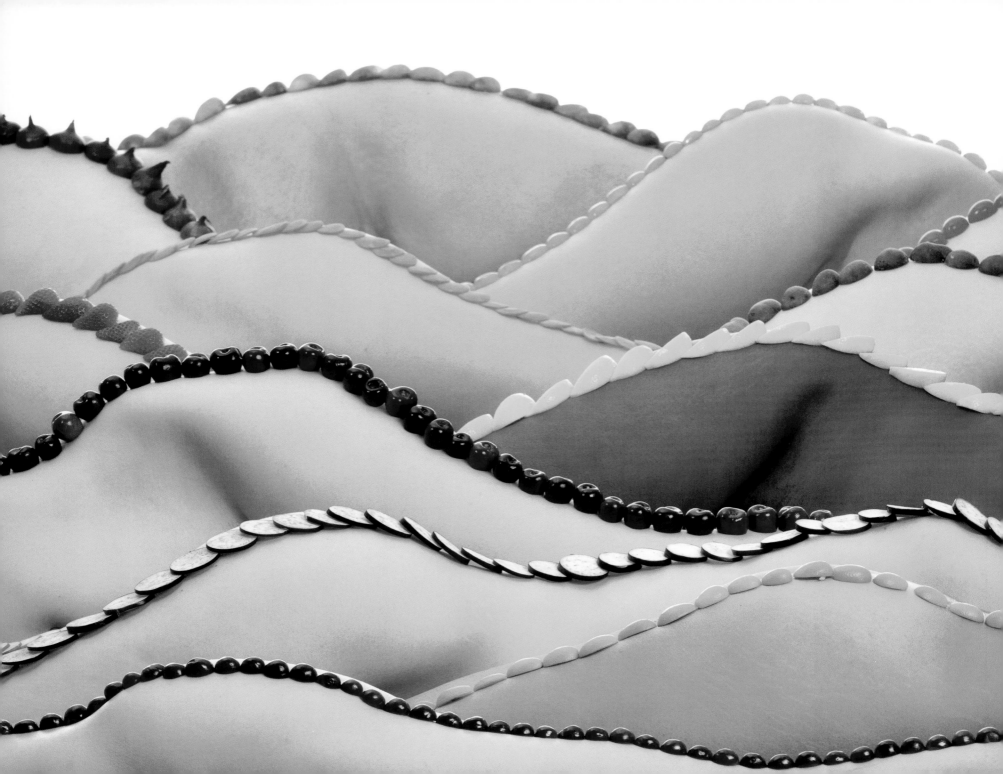

BLENDING FOOD AND FORM

SPUN SUGAR, NAKED BODIES, AND THE MONKFISH'S BELLY

If you had told me twenty years ago that one day I would be creating art by putting food on naked people's bodies, I would have thought you were crazy. After all, I was a sometimes-shy Italian who'd grown up on a farm and aspired to be a chef; I didn't consider myself an artist.

How could I be? I had never gone to art school…in fact, I had barely gone to school at all in Italy. In Seattle, after years of feeling stupid and uneducated when I compared myself to the people around me (who all seemed to have degrees of some type), I earned my G.E.D. But nothing changed and I realized there are many different ways to be smart. Cooking was my opportunity to be smart about something; it was my own personal-growth avenue toward self-discovery and an opportunity for sharing what I'd learned at the knee of an expert.

My mother's ability to produce amazing meals from basic, farm-fresh ingredients always fascinated me. I craved opportunities to spend more time with her in the kitchen, experimenting with different combinations of ingredients and with methods of preparing food. When I moved to the States where my (now ex-) wife and I worked opposite shifts, it

dawned on me what I could do with all the extra time I had on my hands every morning: spend it in the kitchen! But not just any kitchen. I wanted to learn about pastry, so I worked for free in the pastry department of the hotel where I was a cook in the evenings.

At last, I had time to plan, design, and create spectacular desserts—and some that were spectacularly bad. Fortunately, we didn't serve the bad ones, but each failure (and each disaster) taught me something.

Pastry-making is a creative process, I realized, and patience is another necessary ingredient. In my work—which I soon thought of as my art—I challenged myself to try new things on a regular basis. Learning to work with blown sugar fascinated me: the attention to detail it required, the elaborate masterpieces I could create, and the fact that not many other people were working with this process. I set aside some space in my house and began creating art—swans, flower arrangements, a lobster—with only sugar. I donated the finished pieces to the hotel where I worked, and I did this all with my own funds. I was losing money but feeling smart!

Leaves, mushrooms, pinecones, rocks, and branches I found in the woods and on beaches all became materials in my art. I recycled anything I could find and turned it into something functional, like household furniture. My home became a jungle of anything and everything you could ever imagine.

After that, I moved beyond working only with sugar and explored other ways of developing my art. In particular, I wanted to figure out how to communicate ideas I had about food and pleasure and people—and I wanted to use food and pleasure and people as tools to do this.

When I became single again, I joined various creative groups around Seattle. One day, I was invited to a Valentine's Day party. The catch (or the lure!) was that you could not feed yourself—someone else had to put the food in your mouth. People were dressed in sexy, outrageous clothing, and each person had a different type of food to share, such as oysters. I was intrigued by the idea of feeding others and how the experience could be intimate, sensual, and fun—or not.

Inspired, I decided to host a sensual exotic party at my own house, which I'd named *La Baracca dell'Amore* (The Love Shack). The party's rules were very specific: everyone must come with a date; no pants were allowed unless they were very tight, very short, or very shiny; and people were only welcome in the house if they were wearing sensual or sexy clothing. The house was lit only with candles and decorated with different colors of cloth on the ceiling and the edges of the walls. I wanted everything about the evening to be alluring, welcoming, and scented with fragrances of love.

Each room in the house was designated and decorated for a specific purpose: a room with a swing, for example, a snuggly room, and the kitchen, where I had about twenty different kinds of finger foods. But people used more than their fingers to creatively feed each other!

That was the first time I placed food on my chest and had someone eat off it. Even though this experience was thrilling, and it resonated with all my thoughts about food and pleasure and what we need in life, the concept for *La Figa* still didn't occur to me.

I held this party annually, and several years later I met Matt, the photographer of *La Figa*. We've continued to host this party—now called Sedusa Medusa—ever since.

Over the years, Matt and I have worked together on several art projects. Before *La Figa*, one of our most memorable was for Burning Man, the weeklong art festival and experiment in temporary community, held annually in Nevada's Black Rock Desert. With our friend Dan leading the engineering, Matt and I constructed a magnificent twenty-four-foot monkfish covered with more than three thousand CDs overlapping to look like scales on a real fish. Her name was Saturnia, Monkfish Goddess, Queen of Black Rock City. She was motorized, and we could drive across the desert at up to twenty miles per hour. We operated her from a bright red couch in her mouth, and in her belly was a cozy bedroom.

Later on, I got involved with a sensual erotic theatre created by Jeff Hengst. A great artist, Jeff is one of my favorite erotica painters. The theatre, called Little Red Studio, is a showcase for unusual and erotic live performances. My role was to make dessert and feed it to people in a sensual way. For a while, I used a bondage theme and decorated the body with

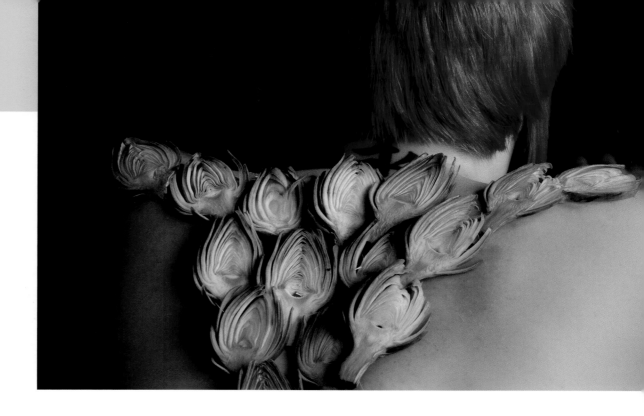

LEARNING TO WORK WITH BLOWN SUGAR
FASCINATED ME: THE ATTENTION TO
DETAIL IT REQUIRED, THE ELABORATE
MASTERPIECES I COULD CREATE, AND
THE FACT THAT NOT MANY OTHER PEOPLE
WERE WORKING WITH THIS PROCESS.

ropes. Over time, I added dessert on the body of my lovely ex-lover, and later I started to create what I now consider to be real art on the body.

My need to create art on the body was becoming more and more urgent, and I also wanted to document my art through photography. The visions in my mind were so vivid—I had to start soon. Matt was studying figurative photography at the time, and he asked me if he could take pictures of my art—talk about great timing. Matt had to present six photos. I loved the idea and was ready for it.

For our first shoot, I envisioned creating the human embodiment of Saturnia, by completely covering a woman's body with cucumbers, like scales on a fish. To be honest, I was quite nervous because I felt like I didn't know what I was doing; everything was in my head and I had no practical knowledge or experience doing it. Once I started to slice those deep green, firm English cucumbers and place them on the body, I calmed down. I was happy. When I saw how beautiful the two were together—the body and the cucumber slices—I got so excited that I was shaking and sweating. A whole new life was revealing itself to me, and I knew this was going to be the best art I would ever create.

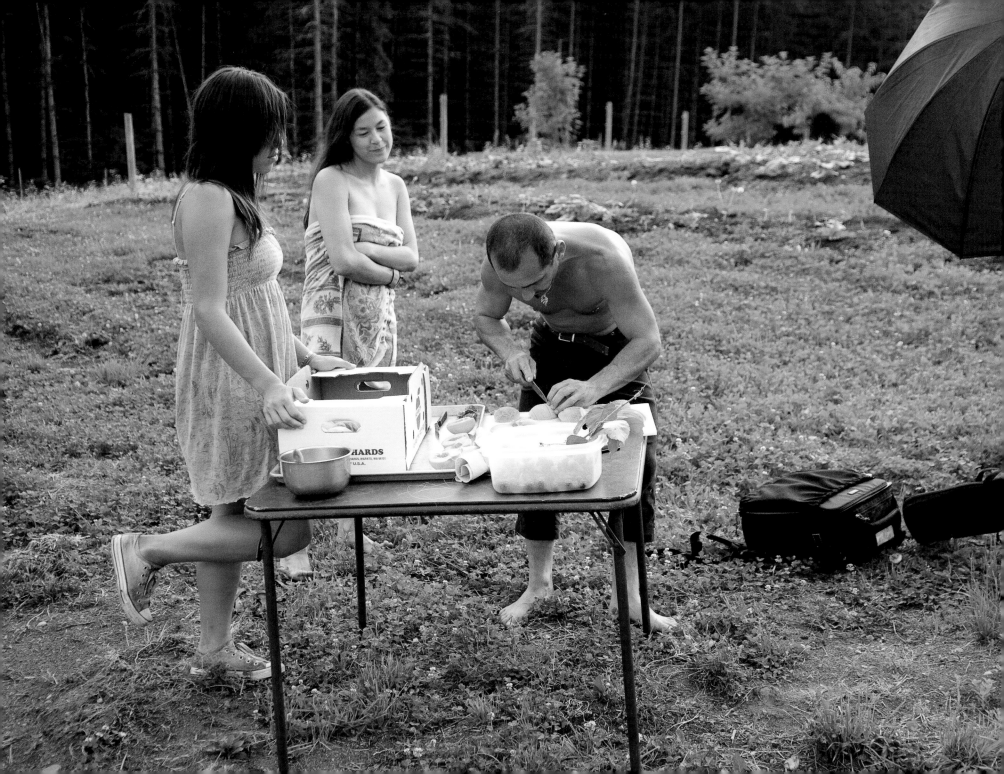

"WHERE ARE THE PEACHES?"

But not just any peaches—I'm talking about the beautiful ones from my childhood in Italy. I appreciate all the wonderful things America has to offer, but when it comes to fresh fruits and vegetables, there is no comparison with my home country—especially the peaches.

Peaches are an exceptional fruit. Once you have enjoyed a great one, it is the standard by which all others are judged. Sadly, most don't measure up. Oh, but when you taste a succulent, perfectly ripe peach, it is truly heaven.

Whenever I see plump, red peaches infused with a brilliant orange color, I can't hold back. I have to pick them up. I love the way they look. I love the way they feel. They are so sexy.

Great peaches always make me think of a beautiful butt. Maybe that's why I like to hold them and spin them in my hands. And, yes, I must confess that I am a big fan of beautiful butts as well.

In Southern Italy, the peaches are amazing. Mmm, there are so many wonderful kinds: small, big, medium, white, green, orange, and bright yellow. They are all my favorites. I prefer them—like butts—in their natural state: picked right from the tree is perfect for me.

When I was about nine years old, my brothers and I had to work on the farm during the summer while most of our friends were free to be kids—playing with each other or going to the beach. We boys were not happy, but it was pointless to complain, so we created our own happiness with fruit. Peaches were one of the most prized pleasures we had.

In July and August, we started our days at 4 a.m. and headed to the tobacco fields. I hated that job because the resin from the tobacco plants is ugly and sticky—so messy and uncomfortable that we wore long sleeves. By 9 or 10 a.m., however, it was too hot to work in the sun with long sleeves, so we moved into the vineyards, where we could go shirtless. But by late morning, it was again so hot that we tried even harder to find an excuse to take a break from any work we were doing in the vineyard.

My favorite excuse was claiming that I had to go to the bathroom. Instead, I went looking for a peach on the adjacent property. This lot was blessed with a variety of fruits including a glorious peach tree filled with my favorite kind of peaches: the bright yellow-skinned ones. God, it was such a treat stealing a couple of them. My mouth is watering right now, as I think about how juicy and soul-satisfying they were.

I remember the first bite, with the peach nectar running down my face and neck, only to be interrupted by my dad yelling, "Aren't you done yet?" I tried to force that yummy goodness into my small mouth as fast as I could. He kept calling for me and I kept stalling. Even though I was racing against time, I remember taking in all that beautiful flesh: from the bright yellow surface, which then became ruby red toward the pit. These colors are as vivid in my mind today as they were all those years ago in Italy. Oh, what a beautiful mess on my face, and what pleasure in my mouth.

Whenever I go home during the summer, I still go to that farm and pick one peach. I sit under the tree located right in a row of grapevines in the vineyard and, when I bite into the peach, my childhood rushes back to me.

I suppose another reason peaches are close to my heart is because of all the memories that come with them. When I was thirteen years old, I hung out with my cousin Antonio (who died just seven years later). As farm kids, we weren't as lucky as the other kids in town who had toys to play with, so we had to make do with what we had. Unfortunately, our creativity often got us into trouble.

Antonio had a neighbor, Uccio, a grumpy old man whose passion in his later years was the two peach trees in his yard. Uccio was very protective of his trees. He also had a dog named Lola, who was small and black and had a big face.

Uccio was the caretaker of this pair of marvelous trees, and, I have to admit, he was a master at producing the perfect peach. To this day, I have never seen any peaches that big and beautiful. Each peach flaunted a stunning blend of colors, including different shades of purple, orange, yellow, red, and even a little white. They were truly magnificent.

One day, Antonio and I were playing Frisbee with an old

lid from a metal paint can. I accidentally threw it too far and it landed in Uccio's yard. We heard him scream that he was going to destroy it and we would never see it again. True to his word, we didn't. We were furious, and we vowed revenge.

The next night, Antonio and I waited until it was very late and the countryside was quiet. We sneaked out of our houses and met at our hiding spot. We were ready to carry out our cleverly devised mission. Antonio's family owned a butcher shop, so he had stolen meat we could use to distract Lola.

Filled with nervous anticipation, we entered Uccio's yard. We tossed the meat to Lola and then climbed the peach trees, being careful not to shake the branches or make any noise.

Even though we were up to no good, it seemed as though the universe was aligning to help us. The moon was full and bright and provided just enough light. The crickets were singing so loudly that they helped drown out our whispers. Within minutes, the true payback began.

We took one bite from every peach on the trees while leaving the fruit still attached to the branch. We worked systematically so that we wouldn't miss a single one. It took us a couple of hours to make our way through all of the peaches—probably about one hundred of them.

By the time we made it home with our bloated stomachs, we were already starting to feel sick; the diarrhea lasted the entire next day.

Two days later, Antonio filled me in on what had happened next. He said he woke up the morning after our escapade to the sound of Uccio screaming at his wife, "Maria,

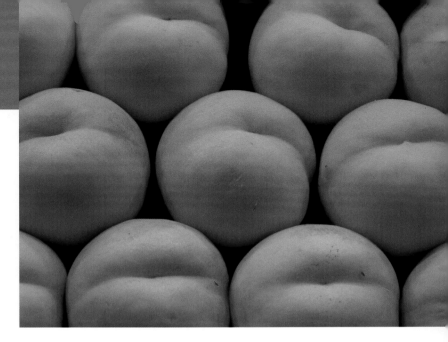

Maria! Look what happened! The devil bit every peach and left them on the trees. Lola, you stupid dog, what were you doing all night, sleeping under the trees?"

Antonio and I both felt terrible. I was sorry that I had done such a bad thing. (Truth be told, I actually liked Uccio a lot.) He died five days later. Antonio and I wondered if we had caused his death. We knew we didn't because he was so old and sick. But still…

Years later, I went to visit his wife, Maria, and we had a beautiful conversation about her husband. She told me many stories about his life and explained how much he liked us. As she reminisced, she spoke about the day he took away our Frisbee. She said he had wanted to give it back, but he felt it was too dangerous for us to play with it since it was made from rusted metal.

She asked me, "Do you remember Uccio's babies? The peach trees. Come, let's go and sit under them."

It was just the two of us; Lola was gone too. She died the day after Uccio did. I looked at a tree and asked if I could have a peach.

"Of course," she answered.

While Maria looked on, I climbed into the tree and took a big bite from one of the peaches without taking it from the branch, of course. Her eyes watered as she gazed at me and a big smile spread across her wrinkled face.

She said, "I knew that. Uccio knew it too. He thought you were brilliant." She went on to explain how he had tried so hard to hold that secret in and not tell our parents because he knew they were violent with their punishments. She said he was very considerate, even protective, of me because he knew I was frequently in trouble and was blamed for nearly everything bad that happened in our town.

I started to cry, and I am crying now too.

Thank you, Uccio.

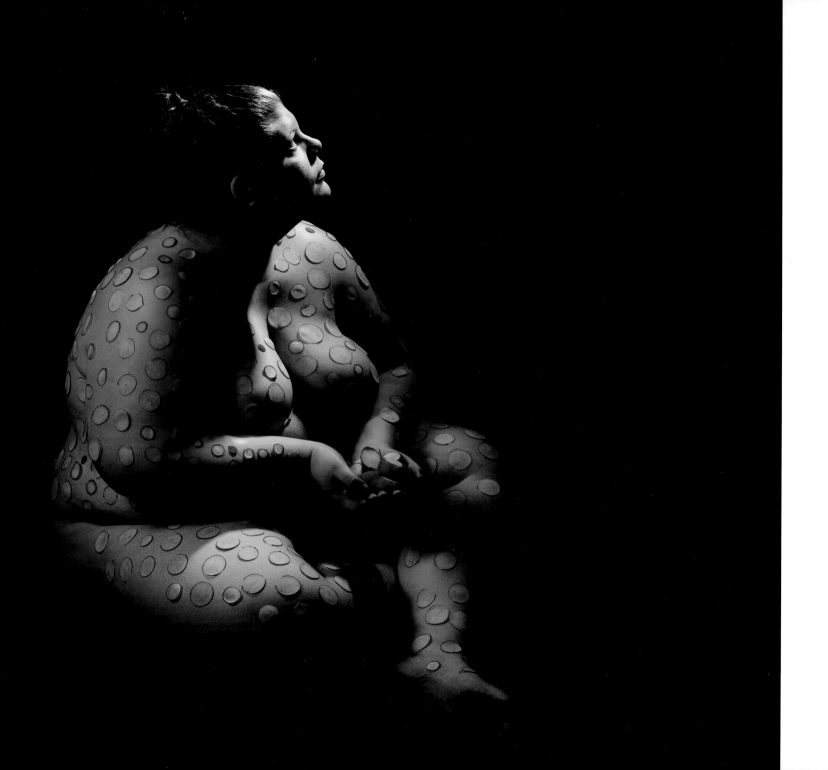

I LOVE PEOPLE. I love food. And I love their shapes. I celebrate all of these with this book.

When I first came up with the idea to put food on people, however, it was all about art, and contrasting the color of the food with the body. At that time, we used female models who were slender and young—women who are typically more comfortable showing their bodies, and so more agreeable to modeling for us.

It wasn't long before I began to search for people whose bodies were not "perfect." The La Figa concept, I realized, is the idea that we can find beauty in everything and everyone around us. I wanted our pictures to accurately convey my message.

As we worked on the book over the next five years, we sharpened our skills at communicating this idea. The result is that the photos in this book now represent a wide range of people—men and women, young and old, skinny and voluptuous, heterosexual and homosexual. More colors. More shapes. More fun.

At one point during this process, I began looking for a very large female model. It took a couple months to find the right woman, but I finally did. She was a goddess in my eyes. She agreed to model, and my excitement grew. So did

my respect for her. The more I got to know her, the more she became beautiful to me. I certainly didn't want to mess up this new friendship by not having the photo shoot go well. (Trying anything new—a recipe, a hobby, a sport—can be risky, and we have occasionally had a photo shoot that flopped.)

I wanted plenty of time to select which fruit or vegetable would contrast well on her creamy, dark skin. So, days before the shoot, I headed to the store to surround myself with produce.

I remember the moment so vividly. I stepped inside the Central Market in Seattle's Shoreline neighborhood and paused so I could bask in the panoramic view of luscious fruits and vegetables. Everything was there: every shape, size, and color. Mentally, I experimented with different produce items on our model's body and rejected one after another. Despite the array of excellent quality food items, nothing was right—nothing was good enough.

Just then, a melon caught my eye. *Perfetto!* Melons are curved and full. So was my model. Melons have sweet and juicy personalities. So did my model. Melons hide their deliciousness inside, yet, with a closer look, it's easy to discover everything they have to offer—something society

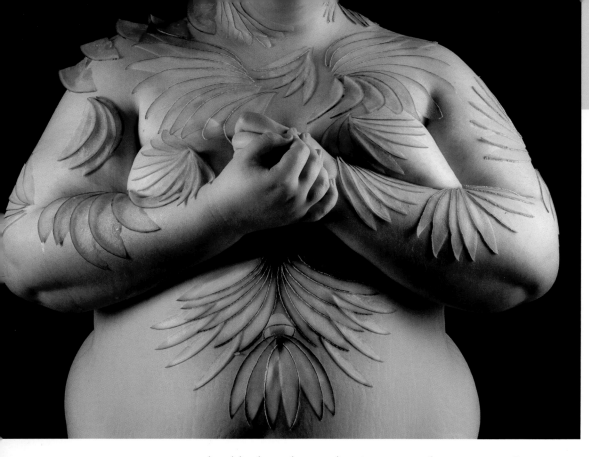

I saw this connection that day and have developed it even more since then. For example, I associate cucumbers and other phallic-shaped produce with tall and skinny people. With cauliflowers, melons, and other round or dense shapes, I think of curvy people. When I see oranges or grapefruits, I think of a woman's breasts with goose bumps. And when I hold a good-sized peach in my hand, I think of a woman's butt—but not a man's. Eggplants are a sexy woman in her forties with hips. Split figs? Well, that is definitely the female genitalia. Berries and grapes are nipples. I could go on and on, and perhaps someday I will.

I have loved working on the *La Figa* book for many reasons. One of its greatest gifts to me is that I discovered how to recognize beauty in so many more people. Now, I look very carefully to find the quality that makes a person pretty or special. I can honestly say I find everyone attractive. When asked, I gladly share my opinions with others so they, too, can be turned on to new definitions of beautiful.

If you pay attention, you'll see that beauty is everywhere. In the produce section of a market, and in the voluptuous person standing next to you in the checkout line.

should take to heart when it comes to large women. I was certainly learning to do this.

That breakthrough moment crystallized for me the relationship between food and people. It was not simply a matter of which food looks great next to someone's skin, or even which food item the model likes to eat. It was much more than that.

The human shape—no matter what it is—is as beautiful and perfect as anything in the vast array of fruits and vegetables I know and love so well. Perhaps we take our shapes from nature, or nature does from us. Either way, we are connected to what we eat through our shapes.

THE HUMAN SHAPE—NO MATTER
WHAT IT IS—IS AS BEAUTIFUL AND
PERFECT AS ANYTHING IN THE VAST
ARRAY OF FRUITS AND VEGETABLES I
KNOW AND LOVE SO WELL.

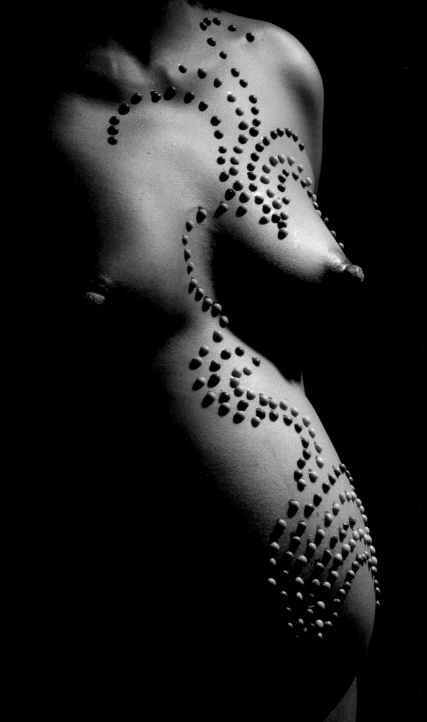

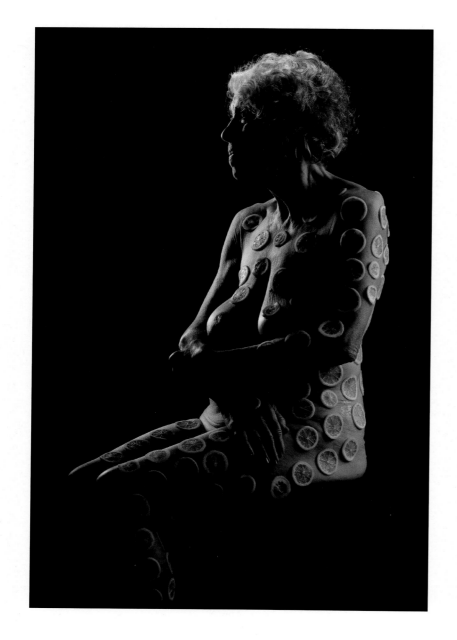
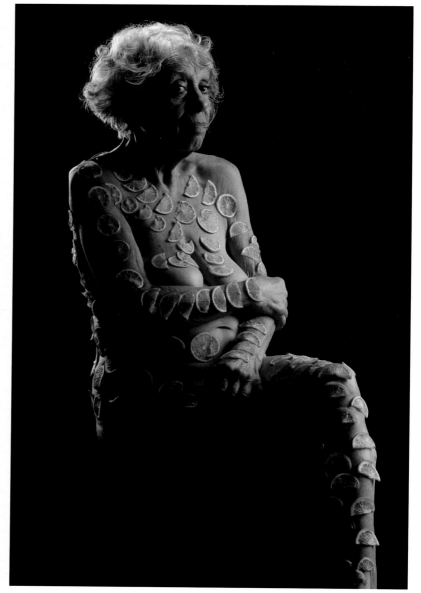

I HAVE LOVED WORKING ON THE "LA FIGA" BOOK
FOR MANY REASONS. ONE OF ITS GREATEST GIFTS
TO ME IS THAT I DISCOVERED HOW TO RECOGNIZE
BEAUTY IN SO MANY MORE PEOPLE.

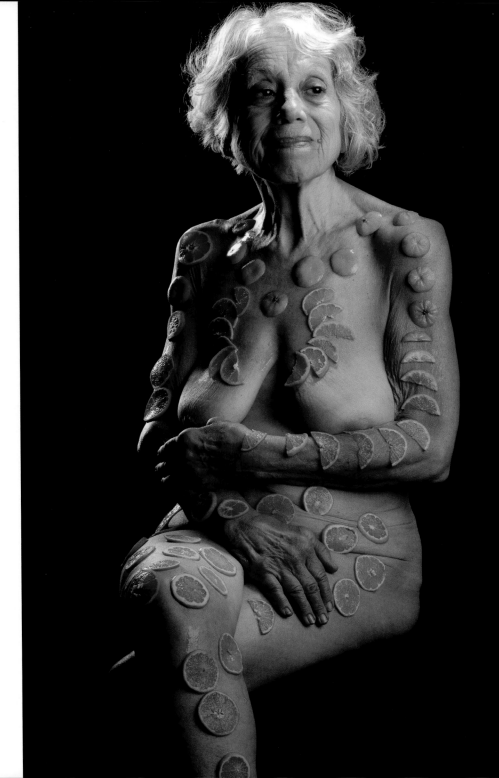

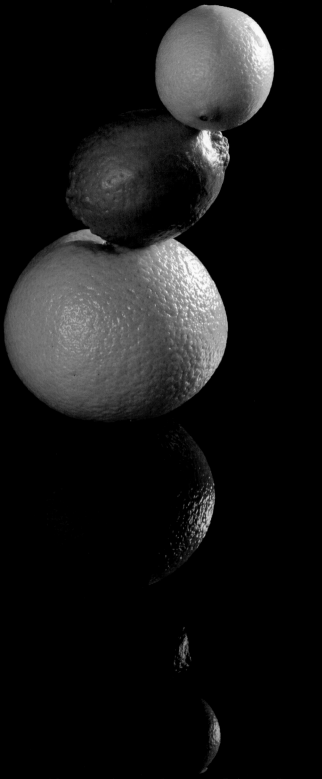

ORANGES

THE COLOR OF LOVE IS ACTUALLY ORANGE—not red, as most people think. Red is strong; it's the color of sex, of roses, of blood. But not of love.

Orange, on the other hand, is warm, sensual, subtle, and seductive. It's respectful, attentive, and present. It's love.

My favorite part of an orange—like my favorite part of people—is the skin. Its beautiful, round form and warm color remind me of firm breasts, with goose bumps. Men and women alike choose citrusy fragrances to enhance their bodies' own natural scents.

CANDIED ORANGE PEELS

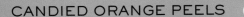

VALENCIA ORANGES FROM SPAIN work well for this recipe. So do blood oranges, with their darker orange skin. I enjoy making this recipe because the idea of not wasting any part of this fruit appeals to me. And, once tasted, the candied orange peels won't soon be forgotten.

Choose at least 4 oranges with a good amount of pulp. With a sharp knife, remove the skin and the white pulp from the orange, making sure no orange flesh is on the pulp. Slice the skin in strips about 1/4-inch wide. Use the meat of the orange for another recipe, such as a salad, or simply snack on it now.

Place the strips in a pot, cover them with cold water, and bring to boil. Let them boil for 1 minute, strain the contents through a colander, and place the strips back in the same pot. Cover the skins again with cold water and bring the liquid to a boil. At the boiling point, strain the peels again and put them back into the same pan, this time with only 1/2-inch of water. Cover the skins above the water's surface with granulated white sugar.

Bring the water to boil a third time, then turn the heat down slightly, and let the mixture gently boil. Watch for the color of the sugar to change slightly to a very light brown. Do not leave the pan unattended. This is a very important step because, if the color becomes too brown, the burned peel will be tough and bitter, and your delicious creation will be ruined.

When the color changes, remove the pan from the heat and strain the peel mixture again. Let it sit until it is well drained.

Arrange the peels in a single layer on a parchment-lined cookie sheet. After they've completely cooled, place the sticky peels in a bowl, add some granulated sugar, and gently fold the peels until they are well coated.

The candied orange peels are now done and deliciously ready to be eaten or fed to someone else. Leaving the strips on the cookie sheet for an additional twenty-four hours, however, allows the air to create a crunchy crust on the surface of the peel, which many people prefer.

Within a day of making this attractive treat, store it in a glass jar and admire the peels' beauty for up to three weeks. Consider your jar of candied orange peels a handy ingredient for seduction and an easy way to share the sensuality of food with friends. Ask your guests to close their eyes, and then enjoy the expressions on their faces as you feed an orange peel to each of them with your fingers.

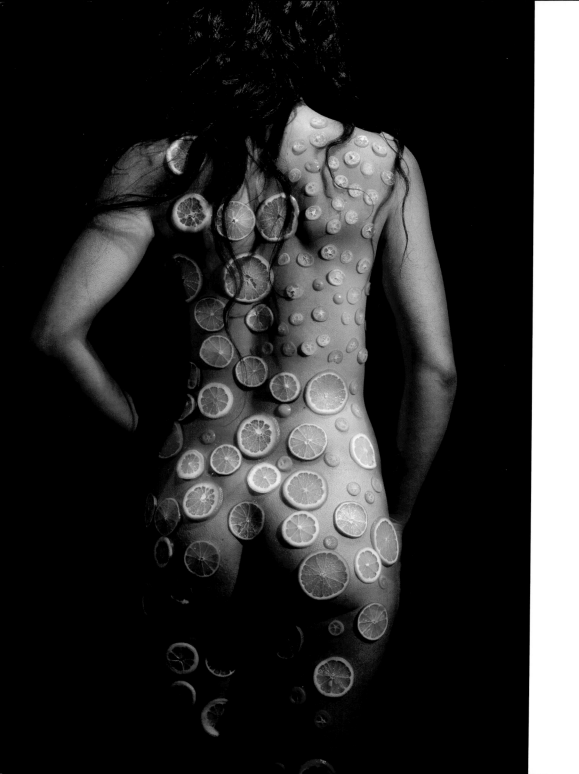
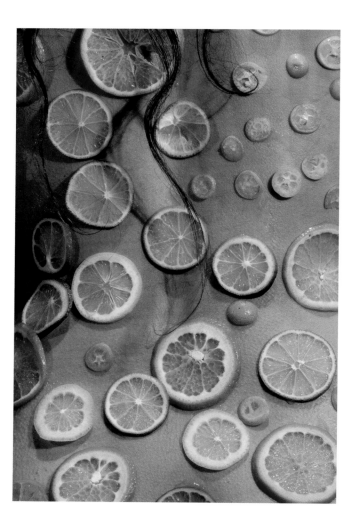

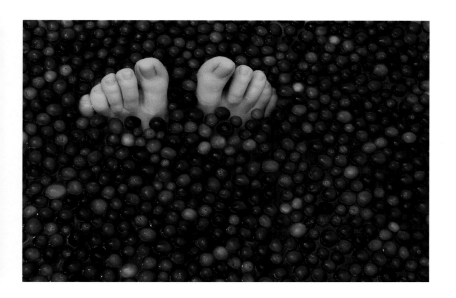

89

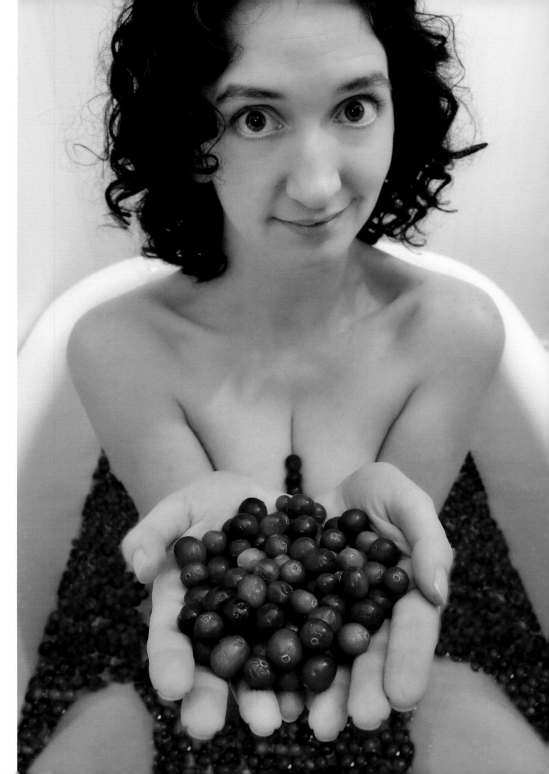

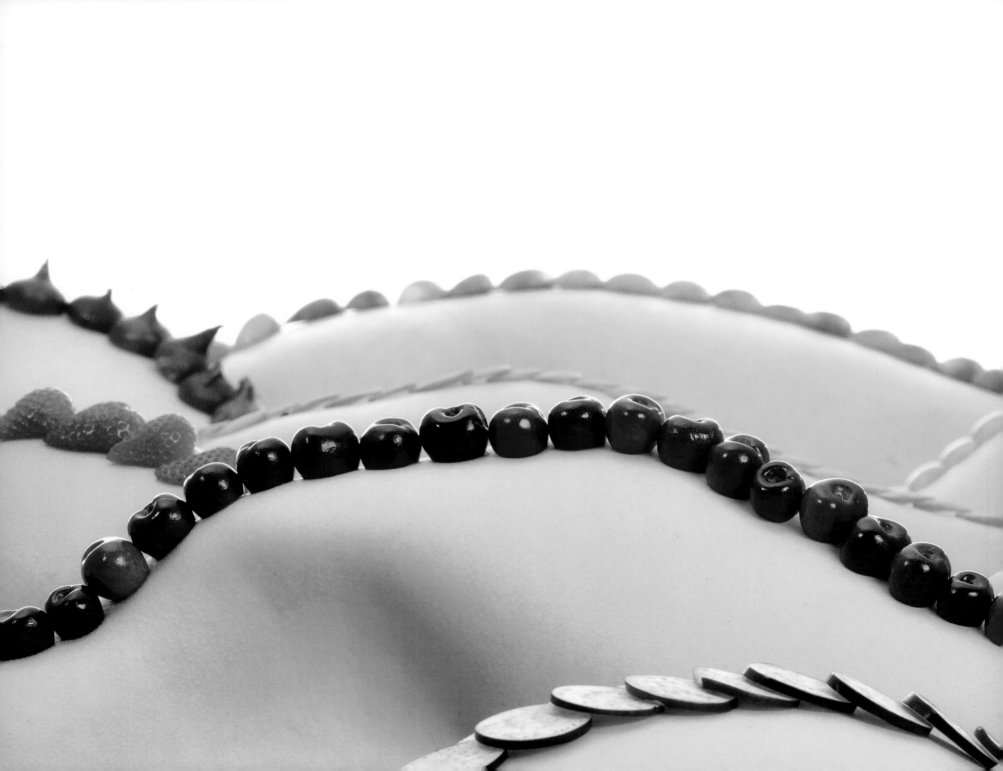

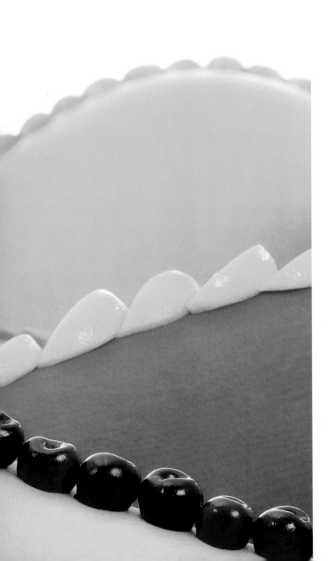

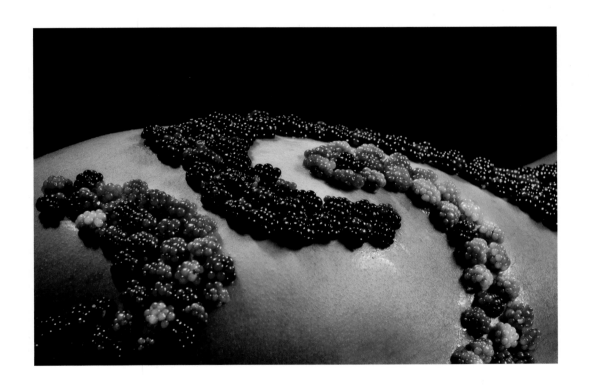

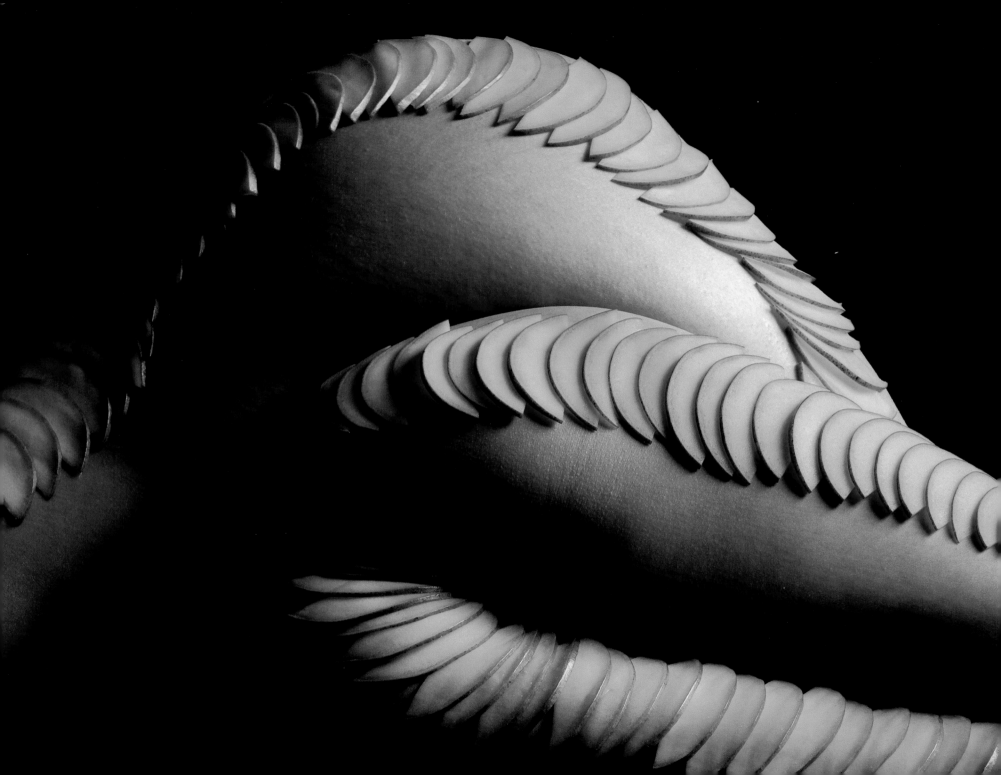

MANGOS

MOST PEOPLE I KNOW LIKE MANGO. It's a beautiful fruit. The first time I tried it, however, I was unimpressed.

At the time, I was a twenty-four-year-old pastry assistant at the Westin Hotel in Seattle. We were using mango fans to decorate dessert plates for a sit-down dinner for one thousand people. While we were working, I heard the pastry chef raving on and on about how his wife could eat mango all day, and he didn't understand it because he totally disliked it. I had never tasted it before, so I decided to try it and, to be honest, it wasn't very good. The color was pretty and it looked great on the white plate next to the cheesecake with red raspberry sauce—but the mango itself was flavorless and a little bitter.

I couldn't understand why we were using it if it didn't have much taste, but I shrugged and decided it must be for decorative purposes only. As the afternoon wore on, I kept thinking about the pastry chef's wife, and I grew curious. I tasted slices from different mangos to find the sweetness I thought I was missing, but I kept coming up with the same bland result. I gave up and didn't really think about it anymore.

About four years later, I was walking with a new friend who I was very attracted to. Actually, it was mutual; we had a little crush on each other. I asked her questions about her favorite ingredients so I could make her a special dinner.

"I *love* mango!" she blurted, and then grinned at me.

I had déjà vu. Here was another woman who loved this fruit that I had found so bland.

When I told her I didn't really care for mango because it didn't have any flavor, she said it was because I had never had a good one. I was skeptical, but she promised that she would find a good one and then surprise me with it in a very special way.

We eventually became lovers. One beautiful summer day, we were in her backyard and she asked if she could blindfold me, and I agreed, of course. I lay flat on my back and she covered my eyes with a silky blue fabric. She gave me very small kisses all over my body, and, once in awhile, I felt the brush of something cold on my skin. It made me jump a bit, and I had no idea what it was. She licked her warm tongue on the area where she had brushed my skin, and made sweet, provocative noises. I could hear her lips and mouth quietly eating something, so I asked—even begged—to know what it was. She wouldn't tell me (the tease!), which made this experience all the more fun and mysterious.

Between the little nibbling kisses with sweet small bites, the gentle brushing of our various body parts, the warm licking, and the soft noises, I was getting turned on and excited. She was driving me crazy. I had promised not to remove the cloth from my eyes, but, oh, I was so tempted. I asked her repeatedly what she was brushing on my body.

She eventually replied, "I'll give you a hint…it is my favorite fruit."

Sadly, I did not remember that her favorite fruit was mango. I had completely erased mango from my brain since I never ate it or used it when cooking.

I named every fruit I could think of, but not the right one.

"I can't believe you don't remember," she said.

I thought she was kidding. I said I was so sorry and that I would do anything for her if she would just kiss me once more on my lips.

"Just one more small kiss," she agreed. I heard her put something in her mouth.

She rubbed my lips until I opened my mouth, and she instructed me to suck whatever she put in my mouth—not bite or chew or swallow. I was beginning to understand what a clever and sensuous woman she was.

That slice of fruit went back and forth many times without leaving our mouths. Eventually she ate it and then asked me to guess again. Still, I could not figure it out. All I could taste was a very sweet juice mixed with her saliva. Whatever it was, I knew it was amazingly tasty, sensual, and intensely sexy.

"Okay, let's try again." She placed the slice in my mouth and told me not to eat it until she said so. Incredibly, she kneeled above me and then relaxed onto my face, with her legs spread and her sex sitting on the fruit that was on my lips.

"Eat it now," she cooed, and I did. It was the most delicious fruit I had ever tasted, especially as it mixed with the flavors of her personal fruit on my lips and tongue. The mystery fruit was a mango, I soon found out. I hadn't recognized it because there was no comparison between it and the one I had eaten at the hotel several years before.

This was the best way to fall in love with the mango, and with her. After that day, mangos became a big part of my life. I use them all the time in appetizers, and they are always everyone's favorite.

Just like sex, mangos are beautiful, sexy, juicy, and messy, but only if you get the perfect mango. Just like people.

My creative and sensuous lover also had a great memory. She held me to my promise to do anything if she would only kiss me one more time and give me a final opportunity to guess the fruit. Her request was that I prepare mango or do something unusual with it in ten different ways. So I did.

They were very creative, very sexy, and very delicious.

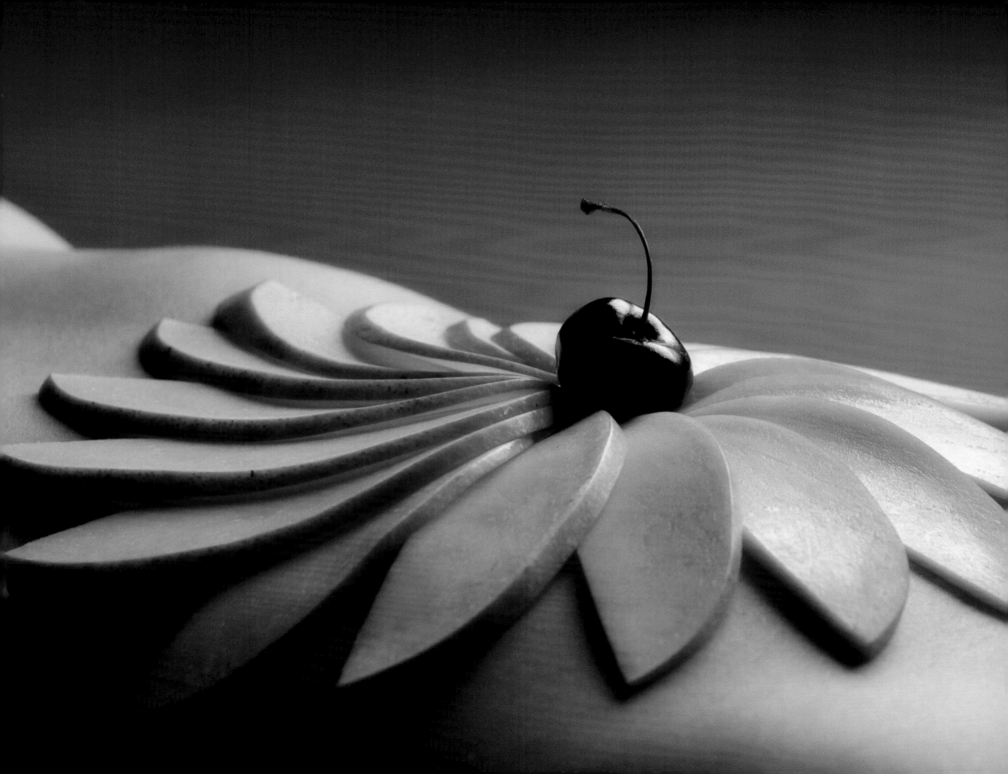

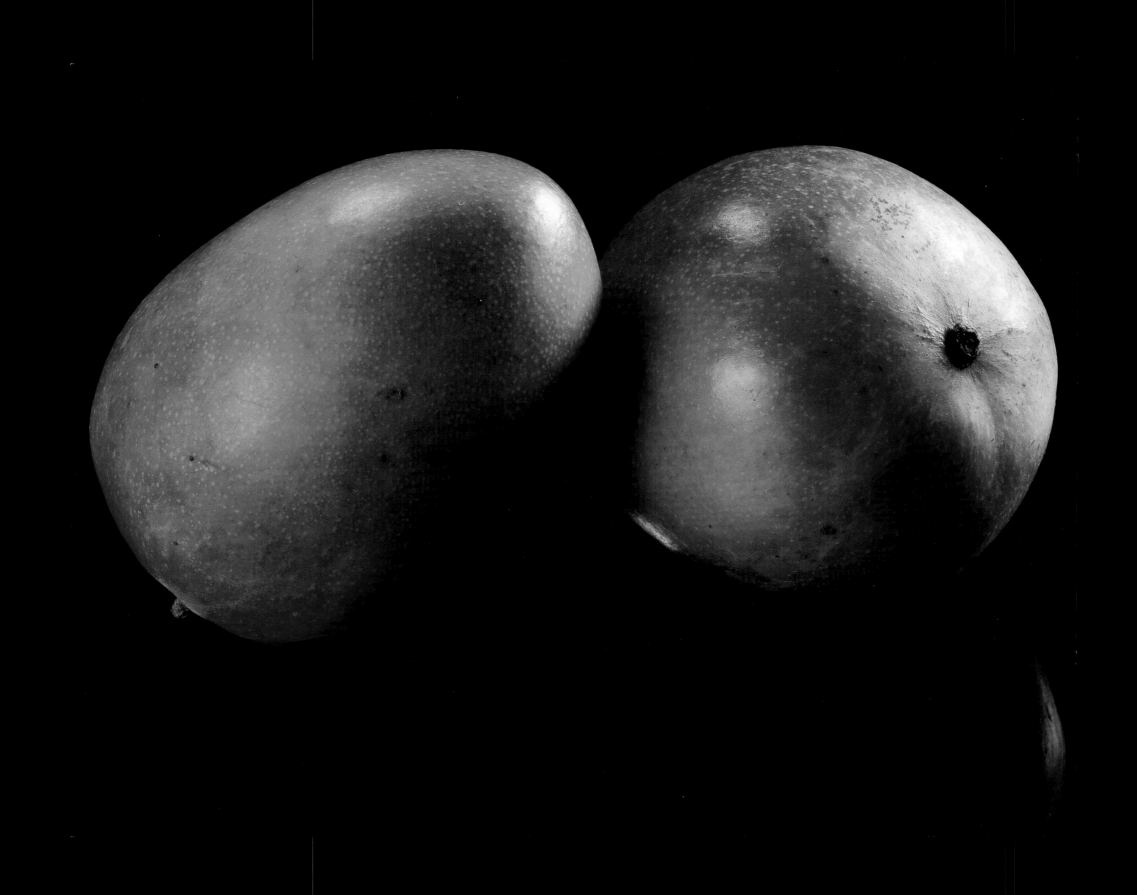

MANGOS

How to Choose a Good Mango:

It takes a little experience to pick a good mango. Most people, like me, learn through trial and error, but you'll definitely master selecting the perfect one.

The primary rule is the mango should not be bruised or too soft. This definitely applies if you're planning to eat it fresh or the same way my lover and I did, which I'll explain in a moment. If the mango is too soft, it will be very stringy and overly sweet. But don't completely avoid soft mangos or throw them away; instead, use them for smoothies or cooked in a sauce.

To pick a mango you plan to eat within the next day or so, hold it in your hand and smell it. If you can smell the flavor and the skin is not too firm, that's the one you want.

Since mangos have a variety of skin colors, do not choose one simply because it is pretty.

Have fun with your perfect mango. If you're with someone special, use your hands to pass the mango back and forth between the two of you a few times. Focus on feeling the curves and the firmness of the fruit. Hold it up to your nose and inhale deeply so you can smell the mango's ripe fragrance. Have the other person do the same. When you're ready, peel off the skin, slice the flesh, and then share it. Get creative. Use your fingers, or perhaps another body part.

If you're looking for a mango recipe to share with other people, try this salsa. I use it regularly in my catering business, and people love it. I have also been known to use it one-on-one, to seduce a new lover.

MANGO SALSA

Choose a large mango that is not too firm or too soft. Make sure it smells good and as a mango should.

Peel it with a peeler or a sharp knife. Slice the flesh into slices between 1/8-inch and 1/4-inch thick, then dice it into cubes of the same size. Add 1/3 cup of red pepper, diced the same way you did the mango. Next, add 1/3 cup or less of red onion, depending on your palate.

Add 1 jalapeño (or a half of one, if you prefer less spice) and dice it as small as possible. Add about 10 to 20 leaves of fresh cilantro—chopped, but not bruised—then a good amount of sea salt to taste, followed by about 1/3 cup of very good Italian or Spanish olive oil, and 2 tablespoons of rice vinegar. If it tastes too sweet to you, add a little fresh lime juice.

Mix all those yummy ingredients in a bowl—but not an aluminum one. Fold it gently, like you're making soft love with someone.

Let it rest for an hour, then put it on fresh baguette toast and feed it to somebody.

That's what I call love.

P.S. This recipe can be used to dress grilled seafood or steaks, chicken breasts, or as a tasty treat on your lover's skin (but avoid sensitive spots).

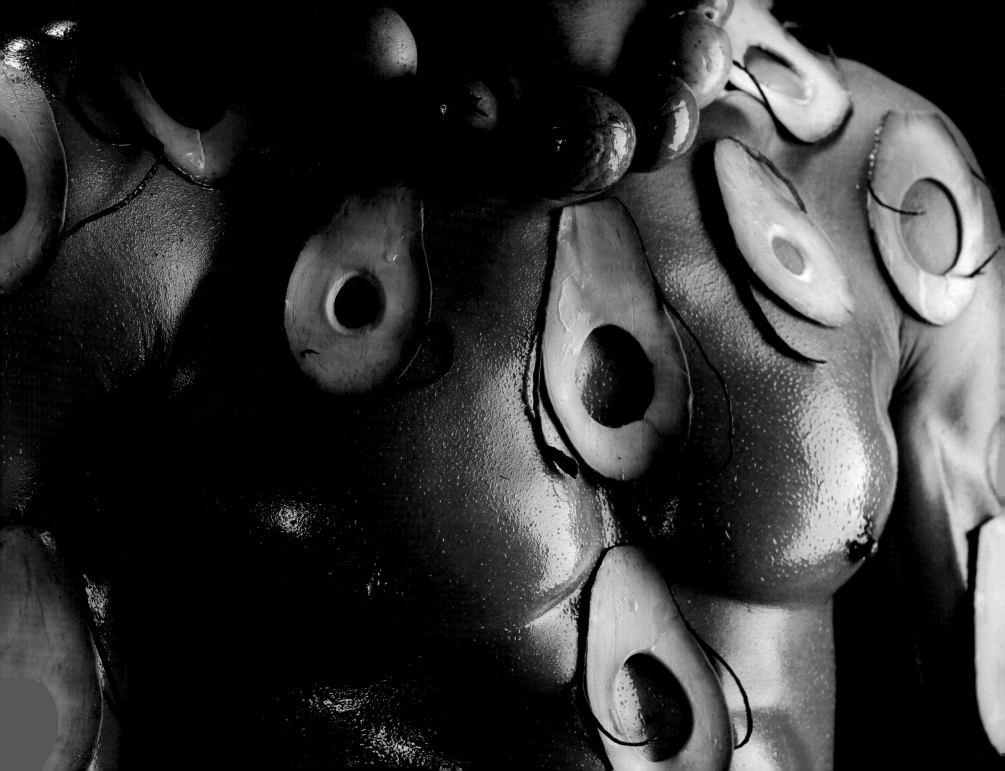

FOOD FOR SENSUAL PLAY

FOOD IS SENSUAL. Life is sensual. People are sensual.

Sensuality is everywhere—I know this because I look for and find it.

Every person is sensual in some way, but some may not see it right away. It just takes a little practice to truly recognize it and then use it in a way that benefits you and others.

Many people have asked me to tell them which foods are sensual. The answer is that every food can be—it's what you *do* with the food that makes it more apparent. And who you do these things with.

Any food with the right person can be sensual as long as you choose something you and your special person find sexy and enticing. Start with food the two of you describe as natural and delicious. Sexy food, I believe, still has the taste nature gave it. There is no better choice than organic food that was grown with love. You can taste the love and care that went into it, and when you share it, your partner will too. Produce you find at a farmer's market is a great choice because you can touch and smell its offerings to your heart's content.

When you go shopping with love and pleasure on your mind, you'll most likely find yourself gravitating toward food that shows the same qualities. If you're planning a sensual meal for your lover and want to surprise her, make sure you know if she has any food allergies or sensitivities. Such foods as chocolate or chili may cause irritation, especially on certain body parts. Trust me on this—I know. Here's a two-word hint: yeast infection. Enough said.

An even better plan is to bring your lover with you on the shopping excursion. View it as a bit of sensual play before the sensual play. You can have lots of fun picking out the food and suggesting unusual and imaginative ways you'll enjoy it together.

When I look at vegetables or fruits at the market, their vibrant colors and sexy shapes catch my eye and make me smile. I imagine how these beautiful fruits and vegetables, when paired with fresh seafood or rich meat, would make people happy. The smell and the feel of food are also a big part of sensuality.

Let's take a peach, for example. Start by looking at its shape and colors. With practice, you'll soon become skilled at picking out the good ones. How do you know if you have a good one? If it looks sensual to you, then it is. It's that simple.

Your second task is to feel it—but don't squish it, of course. Press just hard enough to feel the firmness and the touch of the velvety skin, just like when you touch the skin of another person. I truly believe that fruits and vegetables respond to touch by releasing beautiful aromas for us to breathe in. That's the next step: Slowly bring a piece of food close to your nose and inhale. When I do this, I close my eyes so I can concentrate on the smell.

Paying attention to the sensuality of food creates a special feeling inside that is hard to describe, but it is a good feeling—a deliciously yummy feeling—and it's unusual in a pleasant way.

Noticing the sensuality of food is very similar to how I look at a person or a flower that I find beautiful or attractive. Because I have become so fluent with food, I use those skills and senses to learn about people too, and I often do that by touching or smelling them, or both.

First, I ask if they are single. If they say no, I usually say, "That's okay. I'm not jealous." Then, I ask if I can hug them. About 75 percent of the time people say yes, so I now have their permission to respectfully smell and touch them. I feel their chemistry and learn the way they respond to touch. While this approach might sound silly, it actually works very well. If you decide to try it, you'll be amazed at how many people accept such a request.

The sight, feel, and smell of food are sometimes all it takes to decide if this particular ingredient will be part of your sensual event. Taste, however, is a big part of sensuality but not one you can necessarily determine right away. That's fine—it just adds to the anticipatory mood of the day.

One of the best ways to taste the sensuality of food is when you're eating, which seems obvious, but it's not. There is a difference between eating just to eat, and eating to seduce your senses. Start by breathing in the aroma of a wine that's perfectly paired with your meal. Sip it. Then smell the dish again. Close your eyes and inhale slowly so you can analyze and take in the fresh ingredients and those that are cooked. Take a small bite, and then say something to communicate with that bite of food in your mouth.

"Yummm."

"Breeeeeathe."

"Wowwwwww."

Roll the food around your tongue and move it around in your mouth as you make your sounds. Yes, I know it sounds like a silly thing to do, and when you first try it, you might feel ridiculous, but it is actually a lot of fun, especially if you do it with a romantic date. Many of us say "mmm" or "yum" when we try something we like; I recommend talking directly to that luscious food you're experiencing with all your senses.

As the meal comes to an end, the sensory experience lingers. A beautiful meal creates a beautiful impression on the mind. Your body can now digest the meal and your mind savors the moment. You have shown reverence for the food, and the food has shown it back. When you respect food, it respects you.

If you haven't noticed the sensual character of food, I urge you to discover it. Try my ideas with passion from your heart and mind. And don't just try once. Try as many times as you can. Eventually you will see the sexy qualities of food, and all your future meals will be better. It works the same with people. Sometimes you can see the same person for years and never really notice them, but when you look at them in a different light, you recognize all the wonderful qualities you had never taken the time to appreciate.

Spend a little time looking for the sensual aspects of food, and I guarantee you will become a pro at enjoying the sensual side of life.

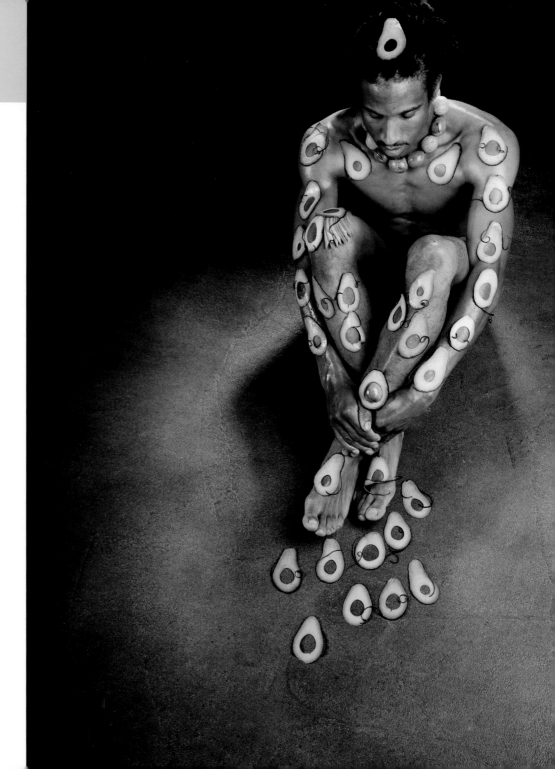

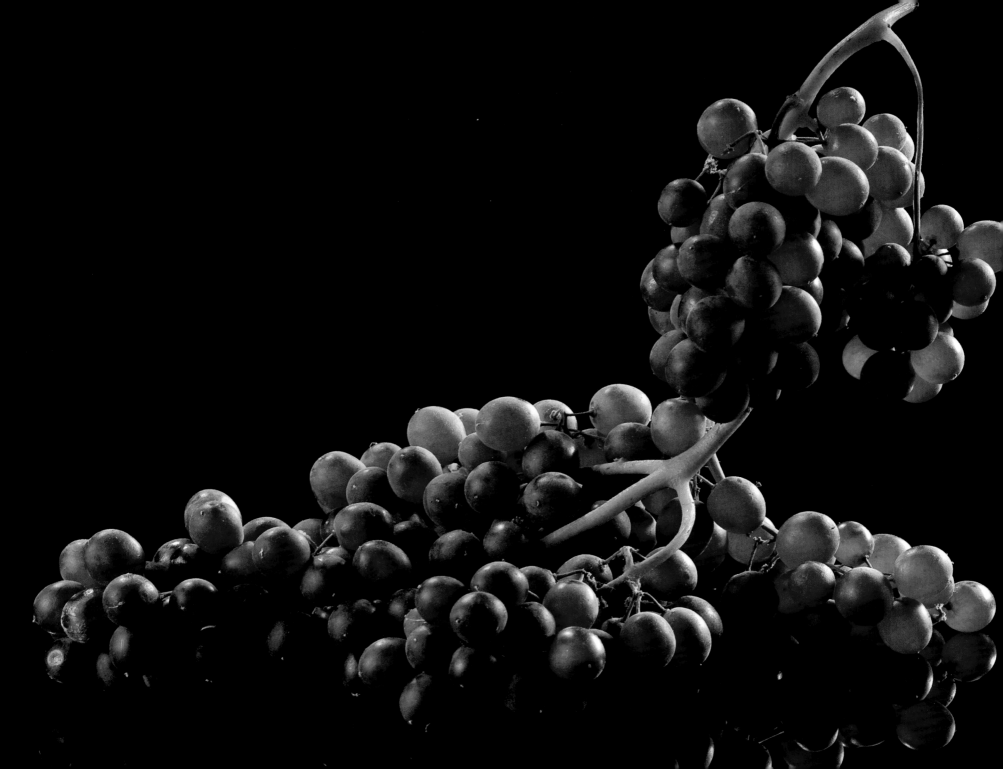

GRAPES

GRAPES ARE ONE OF THOSE FRUITS that are easily eaten on their own...and are even better when you share them. The ancient Romans knew this; they understood the pleasures of parties, food, and love-making. They fed grapes to their lovers in a very seductive way, and we would do well to follow their example.

Try it the next time you come across a perfectly ripe, sweet, beautiful cluster of grapes. Discover enticing alternatives to using simply your hands and mouth when you and your lover feed them to each other.

By incorporating grapes into a recipe, however, we can enjoy their taste and texture more often. They can add a subtle, underlying flavor to a dish, or create a strong, bold presence that gets attention.

A few years ago, I was asked to create a unique New York steak recipe. After working with the result, I discovered many ways to use it with vegetarian and other dishes, and how simply perfect it tastes when spread on a crostini with gorgonzola or goat cheese.

WHOLE GRAPE SAUCE

Purchase 1/2 lb. of concord grapes and 1/2 lb. of green grapes—make sure they're both a seedless variety. Remove the grapes from the stem, then wash and set them aside. Peel, slice, and have a couple of garlic cloves handy.

Place a large sauté pan over high heat. Once the pan is very hot, turn the heat down to a medium setting. Add 1/8 cup of olive oil and the sliced garlic, then immediately place all the grapes in the pan, forming a single layer. Add 1 sprig of fresh rosemary and 1 to 2 teaspoons of fresh thyme and stir for just a few seconds. Let the mixture cook for about 30 seconds, or until you see the garlic starting to turn light brown.

Turn the heat up as high as it will go and immediately add 1 cup of dry white wine, 1/2 cup of port wine, and the zest from half of the peel of a medium-size lemon. Fold the sauce gently. Once the wine is reduced down to about 1/2 cup, add 3 ozs. of thinly sliced butter. After the butter has melted, fold it over the smooth skin of the grapes. Finish the sauce with a pinch or two of good sea salt.

In addition to vegetarian and meat dishes, try using this sauce on desserts and, of course, the human body. You and your partner will feel loved.

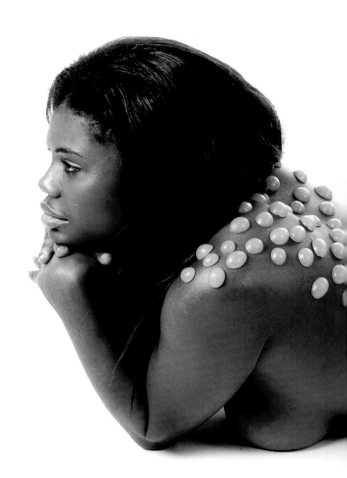

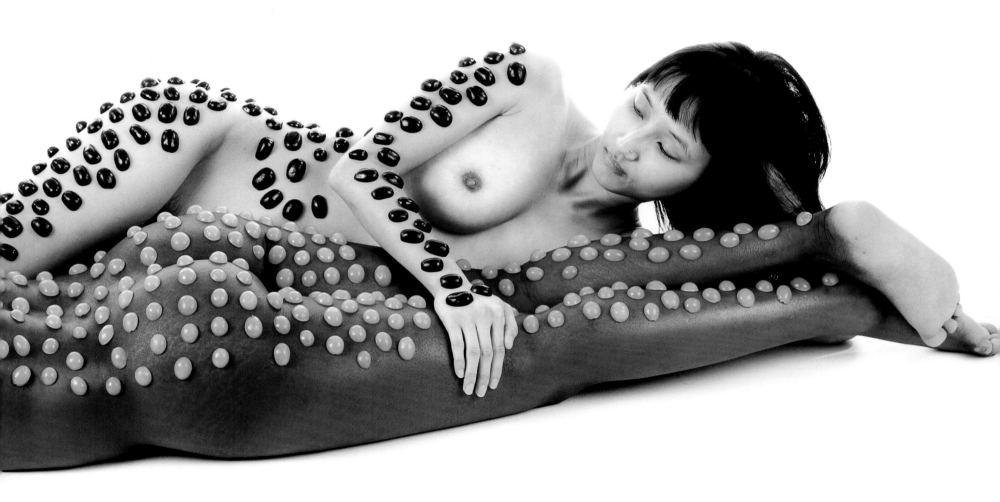

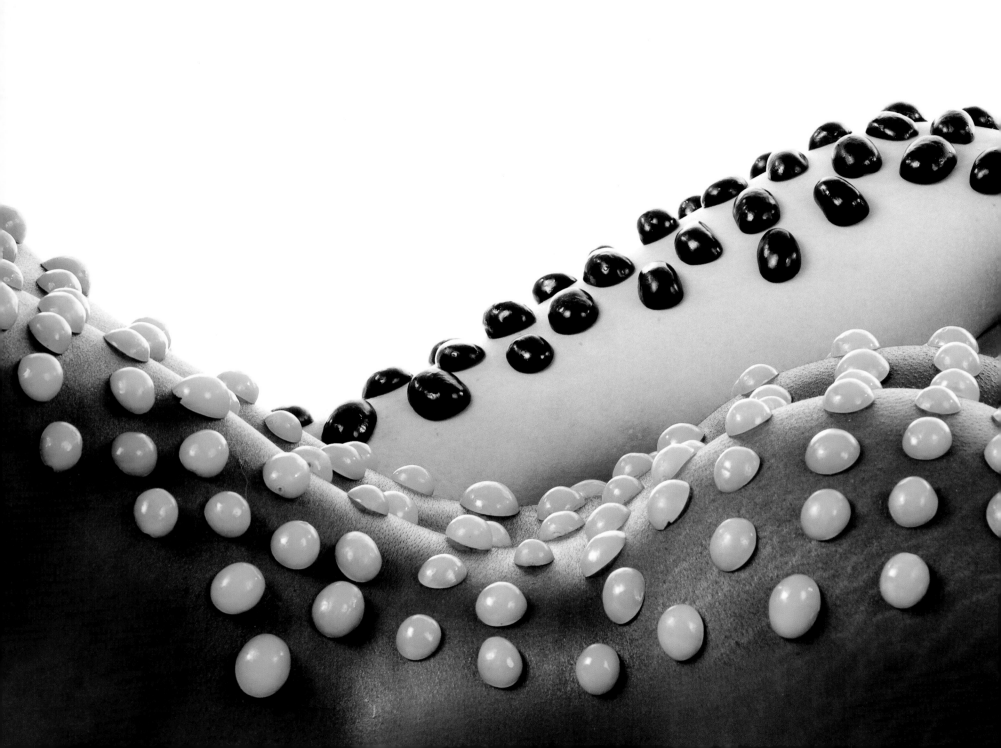

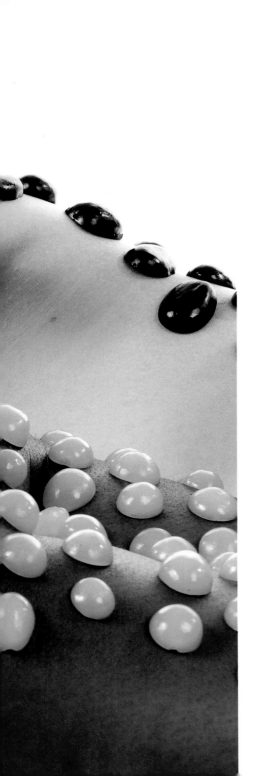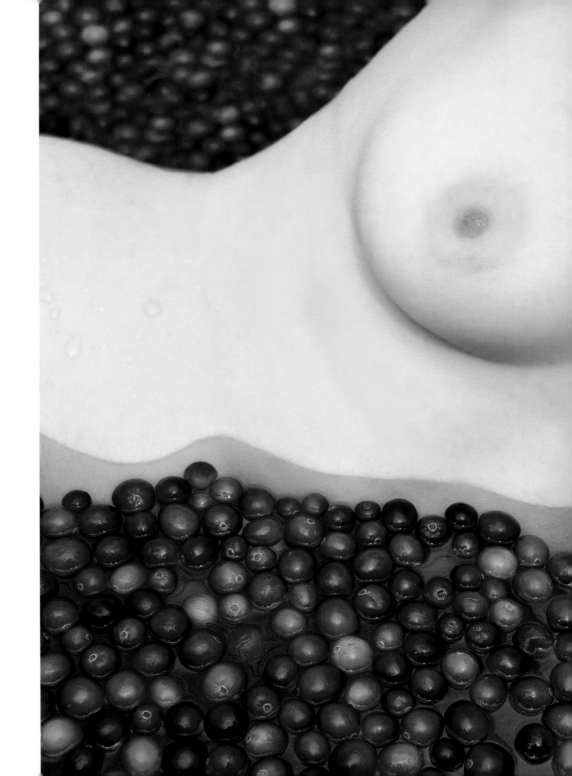

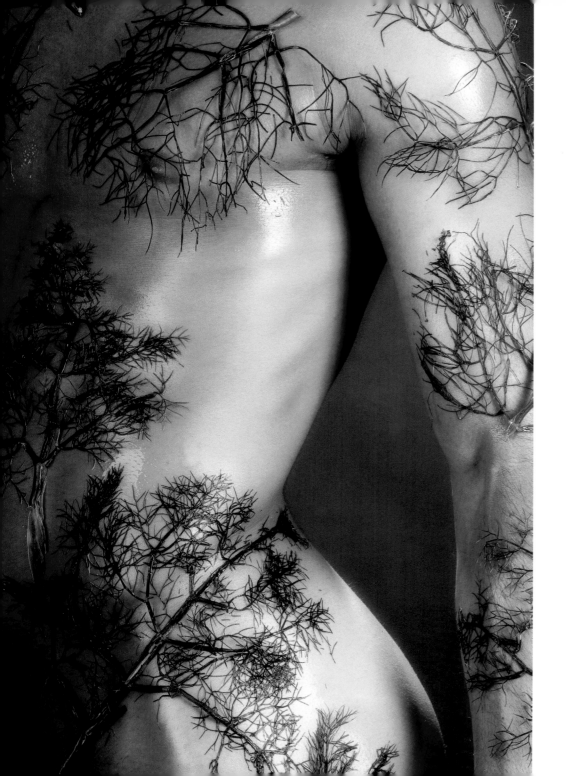

MY GRANDMOTHER USED THE TERM "THE BLESSING OF THE FOOD" WHEN SHE DRIZZLED FRESH, RAW OLIVE OIL OVER SALADS, PASTA DISHES, GRILLED SEAFOOD OR MEAT, OR ANY TYPE OF VEGETABLE.

Il Nettare della Terra: The Nectar of the Earth

MY HERITAGE influences everything about me, so it's not surprising that all the food I cook includes an ingredient from my past or is a variation of a wonderful recipe from my country, my town, or my family.

Centuries ago in Italy, my forefathers began a relationship with olive oil that I continue today in the United States. Consequently, olive oil is more than a staple on my pantry shelf—it's a cornerstone in the foundation of who I am. It's a constant presence in my life as a chef, caterer, artist, and lover.

Yet, even after all these years, the smell of olive oil produces strong childhood memories—some great and others…well, not so great. Either way, olive oil was a key ingredient in my development.

My hometown, Neviano, is set amid orchards and fields and rolling hills in the "boot heel" of southeastern Italy. Like the generations before us, we farmed the land, and it was expected I would carry on this tradition.

One of my earliest memories is of running barefoot through the olive fields. Even as a three-year-old, I was really fast. The giant, century-old olive trees filled with curves and knots looked like imposing statues looming over the land. Undaunted, I tried to climb them, but I was too small to get very far. With tears of frustration on my face, I looked up into the leaves and vowed I would someday explore these fascinating trees and view my world from a lordly perch in the olive branches. Eventually, I did.

As I got older, my wintertime job was to pick olives—an unromantic task, at best, since it's often cold and the work can be very hard on the back. The romantic part comes later, when you get your hands on pure olive oil…and know how to use it.

Like everyone in Italy whose roots stretch deep into the soil, my mother and grandmothers were great cooks. They weren't the only ones to call olive oil *the golden nectar of the earth,* and rightfully so, because it is fundamental to the Italian diet. My grandmother used the term *the blessing of the food* when she drizzled fresh, raw olive oil over salads, pasta dishes, grilled seafood, grilled meat, or any type of grilled, boiled, or raw vegetables. I continue her tradition. Lately, I have replaced butter with olive oil in some of my desserts and savory tarts. The results have been excellent.

This nectar—and sometimes the olives themselves—were essential to many of the breads my family made from the grain we grew. Bread and olive oil, I have realized, are a powerful combination.

The *taralli,* for example, are doughnut-shaped breads made with plenty of olive oil. Yummy and light, we dip this bread in water with olive oil before eating it. We also use olive oil in the making and eating of the *piezzu*—a solid, round bread that keeps fresh and moist for about a week.

My family also made *pucce*, a very popular bread in our Salento region. While the basic dough is similar to that of *piezzu*, *pucce* incorporates more water and a lot of small, cured olives with their pits still inside, which are called *celines*. If you've never tried *pucce*, be careful: you can damage a tooth on an olive pit. It's worth the risk, however, because there are few pleasures as delicious as eating *pucce* when it comes out of the oven and you're wrapped in the steamy aroma of sweet olives. Even at this very moment, when I am far from my kitchen, it's as if I can actually smell *pucce* as it wafts through my memories.

Frisella, another bread, is rolled into a spiral shape about six to eight inches in diameter, then baked two times: first to cook the dough, then to toast it, just like biscotti. This bread is one of my favorites, and, when I think of olive oil, I also think of *frisella* and remember watching my mom prepare and serve it. Breaking off a chunk of this bread, she dipped it in water for a few seconds. Then, with her bare hands, she tore apart a couple of tomatoes and spread their seeds all over the bread. She finished by placing the flesh of the tomato on top and following it with plenty of sea salt and a good amount of olive oil, of course.

God, whenever I eat this bread, I am always so happy—almost as happy as when I make love. The combination of the texture of the bread, the salt, the sweet tomato, and the smell of the golden olive oil gives me the same sensations of euphoria. My relationship with food is as important as my relationship with sex. They are my best friends and the best combination that nature ever created.

Growing up so completely in tune with the earth and its bounty, I had many fantasies as a child that included things from my surroundings. At the time, I did not know what sex was, so I didn't think of these activities as anything sexual... although I certainly understood sensuality on an intuitive level. When I recall all the things I did with olive oil, well, it's clear that the golden nectar of the earth helped lay the groundwork for who I am as an adult.

When I had a cold as a young child, for example, my grandmother spread warm olive oil on my chest when she tucked me into bed at her house.

"Don't touch the olive oil!" she said.

I did anyway, of course. I really liked how smooth my skin felt—even my fingertips were enticing and begging to be touched and stroked.

Well before I reached puberty, I knew about orgasms. I also knew caressing myself after my grandmother coated my chest with olive oil would not be acceptable behavior. That didn't stop me because I loved the smooth sensation of touching my body with olive-oil-coated fingers. After I was done, I got up from bed and, without making any noise, added more olive oil to my chest so my grandmother would not find out I was touching the oil and myself. Oh, and I cleaned my hand too.

One day, I got caught. My grandmother came to me, showing me my underwear.

"Tiberio, why is your underwear oily?"

"I don't know," I mumbled, very embarrassed. So embarrassed, in fact, I ran home to my parents' house, which was a few blocks away. For a while, I tried to avoid my grandmother because of my deep shame. Nonetheless, the lure of the olive oil on my skin was too much. I didn't stop touching myself—I just got smarter, and removed my underwear first, then used my knees to keep the sheets elevated.

This was my sole source of pleasure for quite a while. I even had a few little bottles of olive oil hidden in the dirt in many different places around our family's vineyard.

I can attest that, as a sexual lubricant, olive oil is great. It smells better and is healthier for our bodies than synthetic products.

As a massage oil, the golden nectar of the earth can't be beat. The skin warms and releases a wonderful smell. On top of that, you can add kisses and licks, if you're giving a sensual massage to the special person in your life. I'm frequently asked how to use olive oil to do this. Here's my advice: Imagine you and your lover are in a snowbound cabin in the wintertime, and the only heat is from the fireplace or whatever the two of you create together. Your lover is lying down on his or her belly, and you start by rubbing warm olive oil into the back, shoulders, butt, and legs of your companion. When you're both ready, have the recipient of this massage roll over so you can spread the oil around the front side of the body. Then, using your naked body as well as your hands, slowly move up and down, side to side, and then in a circle. The two of you will grow warmer and warmer from the friction created by your bodies and with the olive oil serving as the perfect lubricant. From there, the rest is up to you.

Olive oil brings together food and sex for nourishment and enjoyment. Food is life and sex is life. Both provide pleasure.

And if you've ever wondered why Italian people have such wonderful skin and hair, I believe olive oil deserves the credit. It is a wonderful hairstyling product. I place a small amount in my hand and brush it through my hair to get shine and softness. Because it is 100 percent natural, it's good for our hair.

I recommend you discover the wonders of olive oil beyond the spaghetti dinner and even beyond the kitchen. The sensation, the smell, and the wonderful taste will stay with you—and create memories you'll want to revisit over and over again.

Use good olive oil liberally and enjoy *il nettare della terra*, the nectar of the earth.

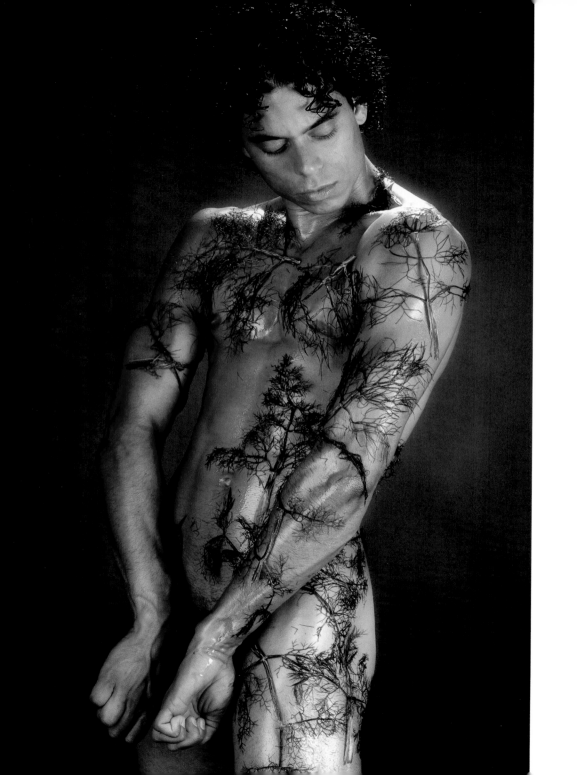

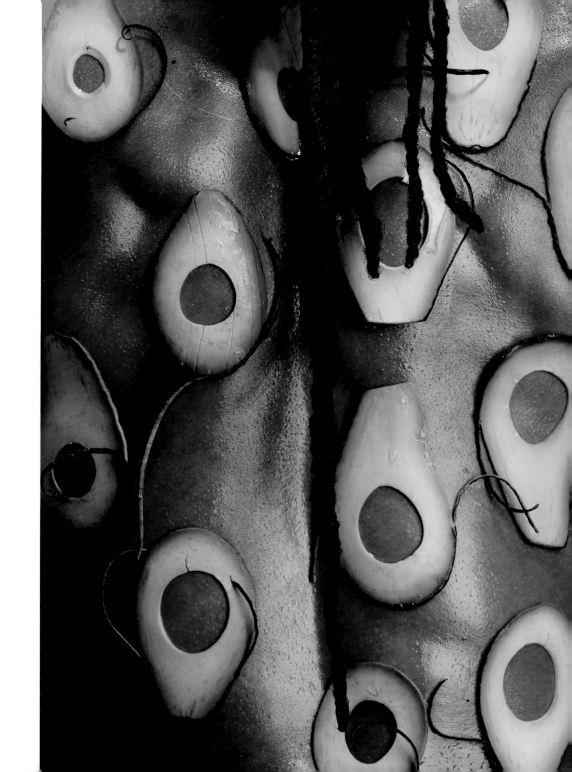

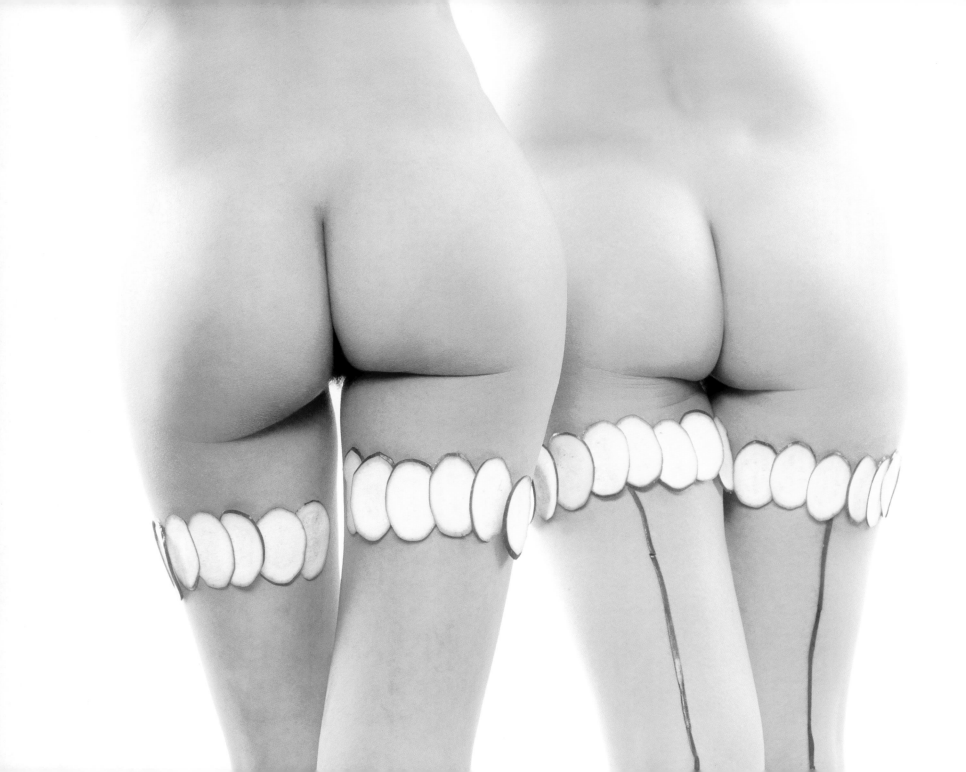

HOW TO FLIRT, SEATTLE-ITALIAN STYLE

FLIRTING IS TRULY AN ART. While some people are naturally better at it than others, it's also a learned skill, thus practice makes perfect. Your personality type, level of confidence, and culture might also contribute to your level of flirting success.

I must admit that, being Italian, I'm wired for flirting. In fact, it's probably one of my best talents. Why? Because the competition for women in Italy is fierce. You need to have "game" in order to triumph over the other men and get the girl. By necessity, Italian men learn early on how to pursue women. Their eyes and posture, how they wear their clothes, their overt charm, and their ability to communicate desire all create a magnetic energy. Here in the United States, I have the added appeal of an Italian accent. Let's be honest, being a genuine Italian in America gives me a natural advantage.

For some people, flirting is difficult because they have been rejected in the past. For some, it is quite impossible because they are way too shy. Others have stupid lines. Some need to be drunk to work up the courage. (Unfortunately, they usually don't realize how drunk they are, although the person they're trying to flirt with does. My advice: don't look for false courage by overindulging.)

There are many ways to flirt. For a man, simply kissing a woman's hand will get her attention. Women can try shaking a man's hand and looking him straight in the eye, then say something flattering about his face, his eyes—a compliment about his physical appearance or presence.

There are other ways to get a person's attention. Try sending a note. Making eye contact often works, especially if you hold their gaze a little longer than they're expecting. Tell them you love their name or you love the fragrance of their perfume. Or say to that person, "You are the best thing to happen to me today." Or simply, "You are so beautiful." Ask questions gently: "Can I give you a hug?" or "Why are you so beautiful?"

My favorite way to flirt with someone who is super shy is to look into her eyes, keep smiling, then look away and back at her eyes again. Repeat this a few times in a natural, leisurely way. Try it—it works wonders.

The No. 1 rule in flirting is to make sure you *really* mean it. If it's fake or contrived, it will not work. When I flirt, I am always honest and that is why I enjoy success. The key is to find a quality that you find attractive in that person. That way, you are both complimentary and honest. Be truly genuine no matter which flirting tactic you use.

If I am very attracted to someone, even I get nervous. So I will simply ask, "Can I flirt with you?" This method works surprisingly well because most people aren't expecting such a disarming approach.

When it comes to touch, a woman can get away with a lot more than a man; it's important to keep that in mind. Men just have to look a little harder for situations where it is appropriate to touch her, and they do exist: holding her hand when crossing a busy street or escorting her (offering your arm to her or putting your hand gently in the small of her back) as you guide her to a seat or a table. Always be on the lookout for anything that needs fixing or adjusting, such as a collar that is out of place or a strand of hair in her face. In this flirting stage, it is important to remember to use very slow, gentle touches.

When people see me flirting, a lot of them ask me how I do it, but it's just part of who I am. Trust me, there are many times I don't even realize I'm doing it until someone says, "You're such a flirt!"

It may not come as easily to you, and so you believe you cannot flirt because it is too hard for you or it's not your style. My advice is to have an open mind and practice, practice, practice. Even though I say flirting is an art, it is just as much about skill as natural talent. I am an accomplished chef, but I had to reach this level of expertise through years of practice and learning from many teachers.

You can do the same if you wish to develop your flirting skills. Ask a friend who is good at flirting to teach you. He or she will probably be flattered you asked. I always am when friends have asked me to give them a little help. The first time, I didn't know what to teach; it wasn't as if I had taught a Flirting 101 class. We started by practicing and role playing. It turned out to be so much fun—and very funny too.

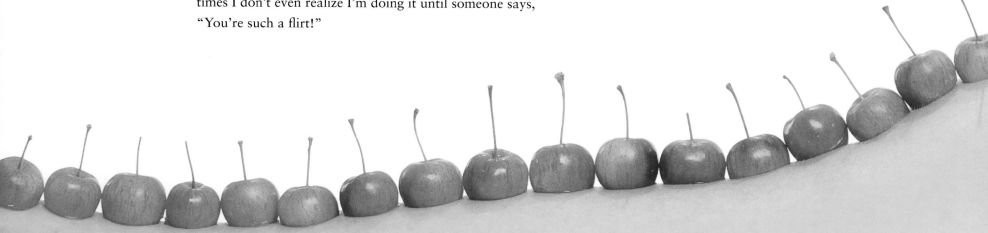

Try these techniques and, sooner or later, someone will flirt back. Once you gain a little confidence, you will see how simple it can be. Keep your perspective by remembering that flirting is just like life: Some people are nice and some people are not so nice. If a person doesn't receive your flirting well, don't take it personally—maybe they are already occupied with someone else. Don't forget to check the ring finger.

Have fun flirting. Do so with true honesty and you will greatly increase your chances of a warm reception. I blow you a good-luck kiss.

Ciao.

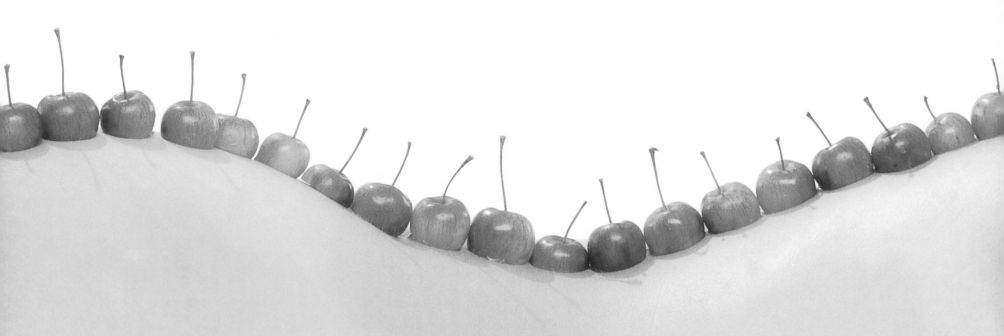

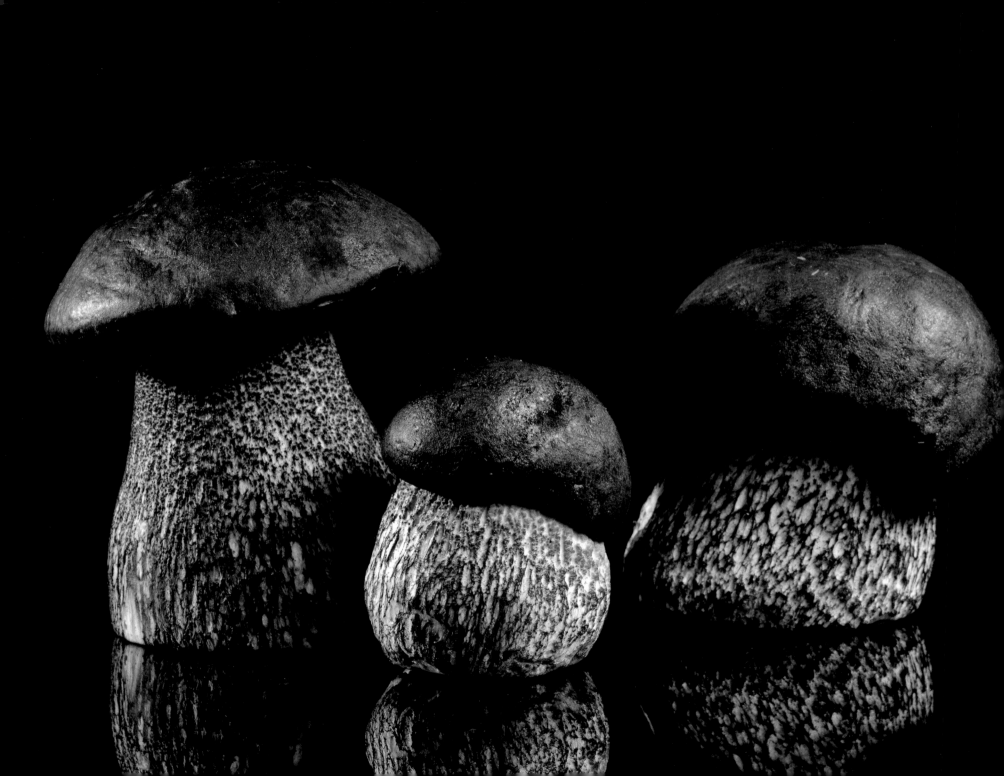

MUSHROOMS

IN THE AUTUMN, mushrooms are perennially my favorite ingredient. Their lush curves, their earthy smell, their subtle colors—what is not to love?

The best part of cooking with mushrooms, however, is foraging for them. A mushroom-hunting day is a much-anticipated opportunity to hop in my car, leave the city, and drive to the mountains. Climbing and hiking provide exercise, and the fresh air stimulates my senses. Discovering a perfect mushroom—or several of them—is like finding treasure. I could spend my entire day there, breathing in the scents of the rich, damp earth and the perfume of the trees. Once I'm finally on the road again, I'm eager to start cooking, and I vow to do justice to this gift that nature has shared with me that day.

Whether I'm in the mountains or at the market, I take extra time to find the type of mushroom I need for a particular recipe. Most good markets carry a few standard varieties, so it can be difficult—but always worth it—to find one of my more unusual favorites. Chanterelles, angel wings, bear's heads, lobsters, porcinis, morels, trumpets, and chicken of the woods are all on my list. One of my favorite mushrooms from the bolete family, however, proudly stands head and shoulders above the rest: the porcini, known as the king bolete.

GRILLED PORCINI MUSHROOMS

USE PORCINI MUSHROOMS to best experience this recipe, and be sure to select large, firm ones. Soft mushrooms will stick to the grill, fall apart, and not satisfy you.

Cut the mushrooms lengthwise into 1/2-inch to 3/4-inch slices or, if a mushroom is not as large as its brothers, cut it in half. Brush both sides of the slices with good olive oil and place the strips on a grill preheated to a high temperature of at least 400°F. Let the strips sit for 3 to 5 minutes and make sure the mushrooms' flesh receives the distinctive black stripe markings from your grill.

Gently flip each slice and grill it as you did the first side, but for a shorter length of time. You should also sprinkle this second side with a good amount of sea salt.

Remove the mushrooms from the grill, place them in a dish in a single layer, and set them aside for a few minutes. Slice a baguette, brush it with oil, and grill it for a couple minutes so both sides are light brown.

Place a slice of mushroom over the bread and eat it. If you like to experiment, squirt a few drops of lemon juice on the mushroom slices, or, for a more intense taste, add a thin slice of Italian gorgonzola.

You'll now discover the true value and pleasure of the treasure you can find in the woods.

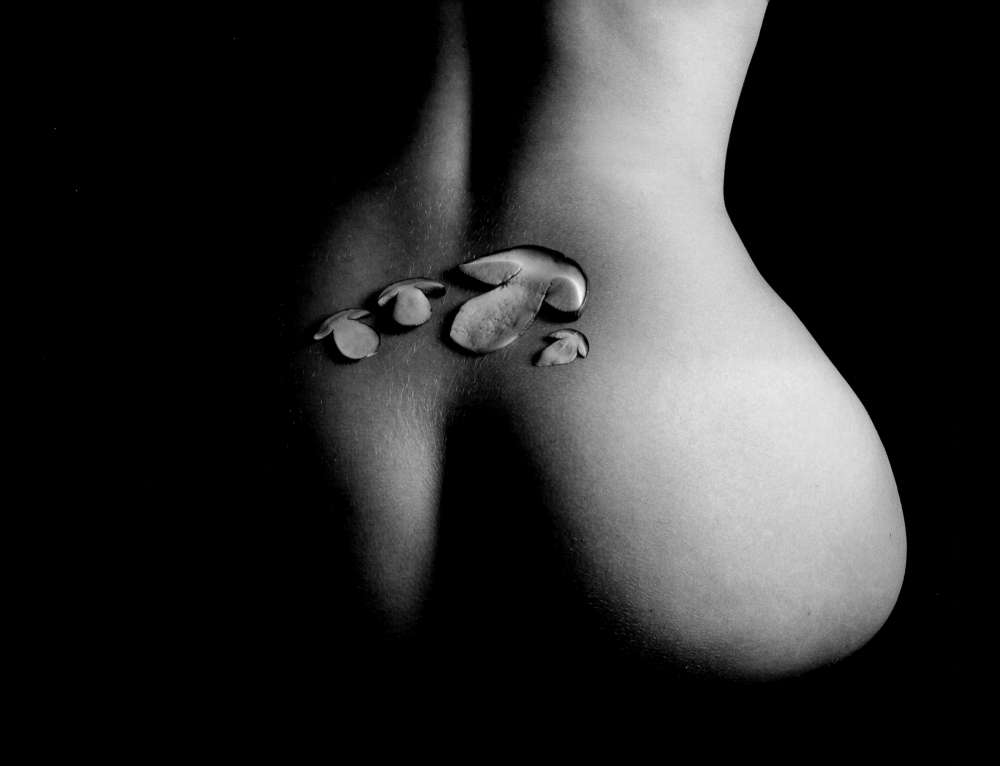

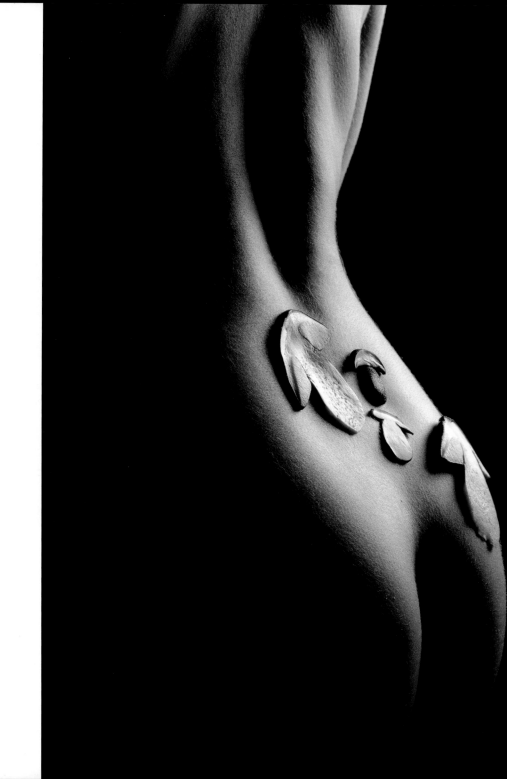

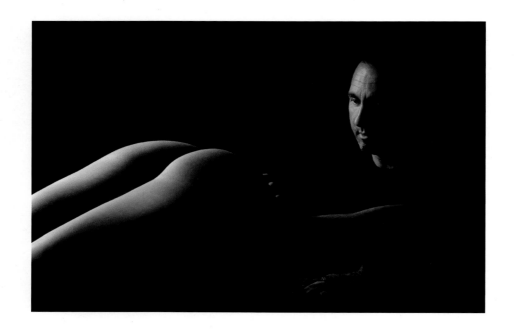

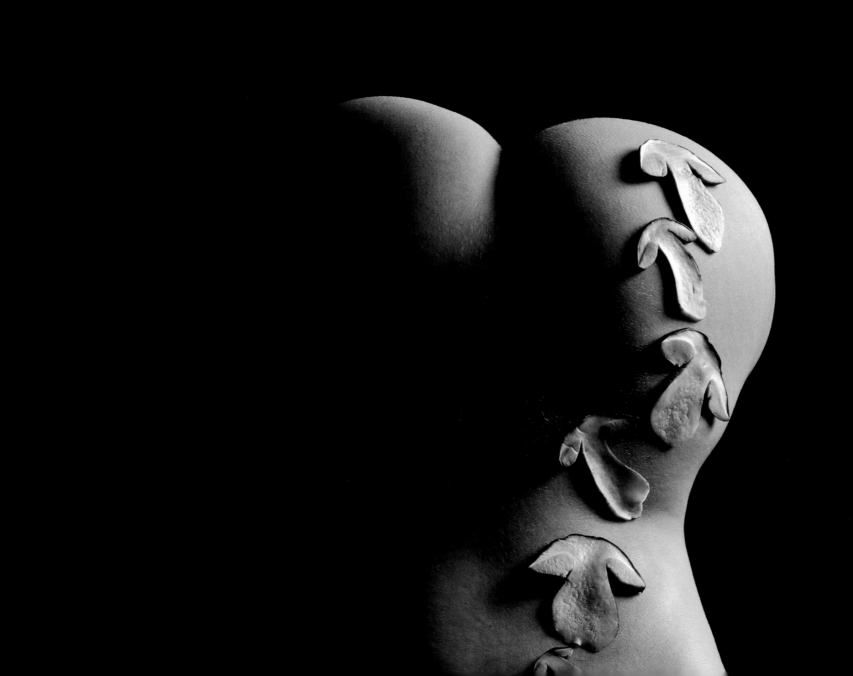

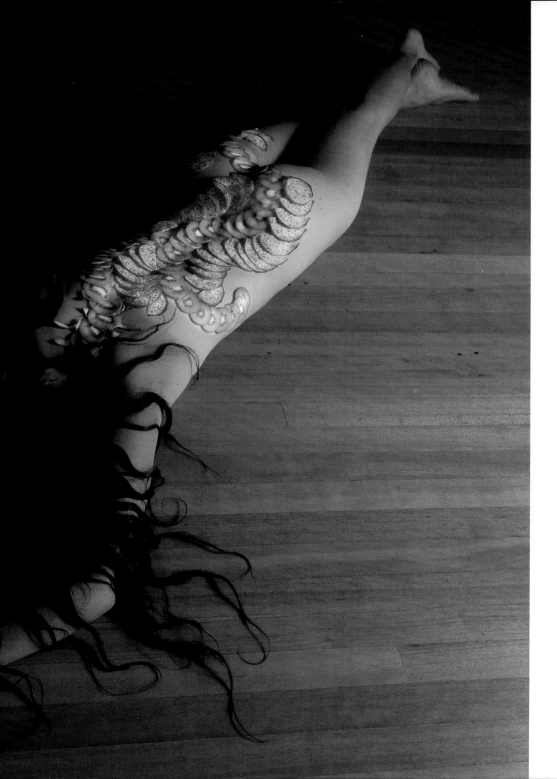

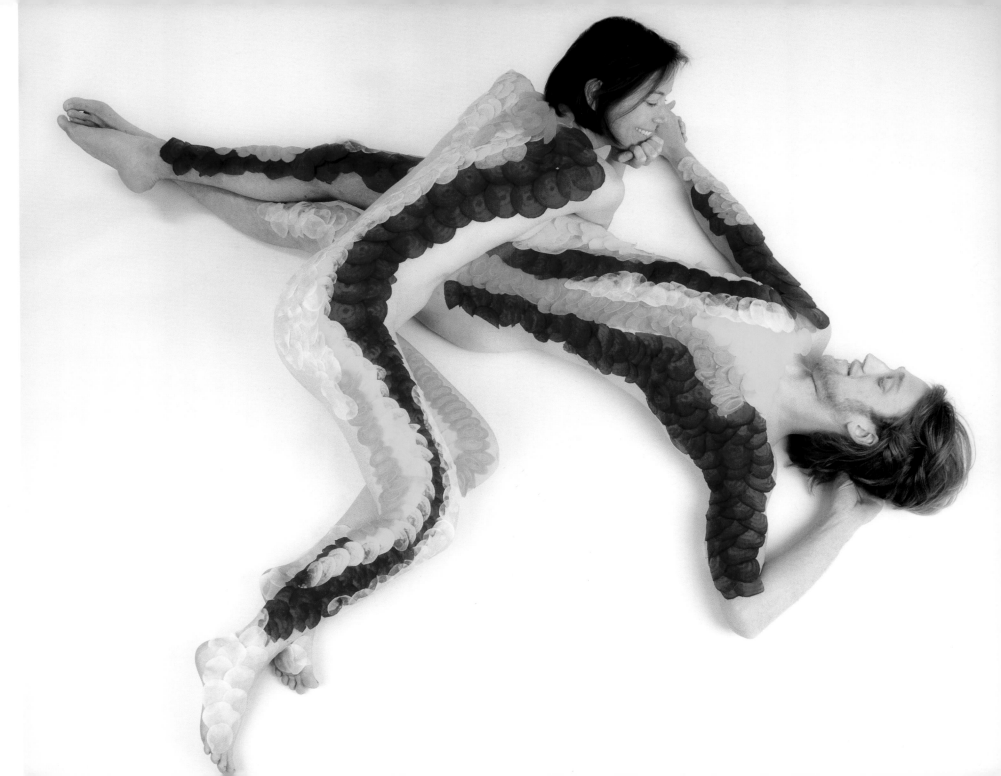

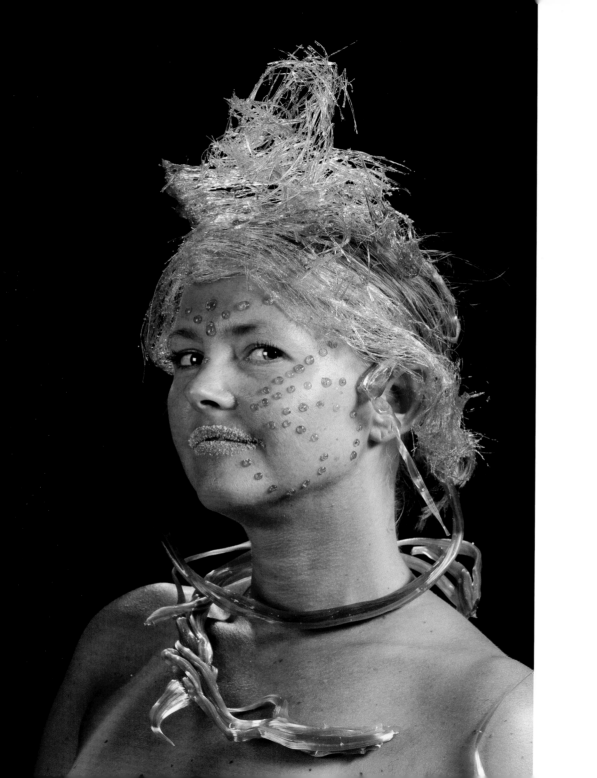

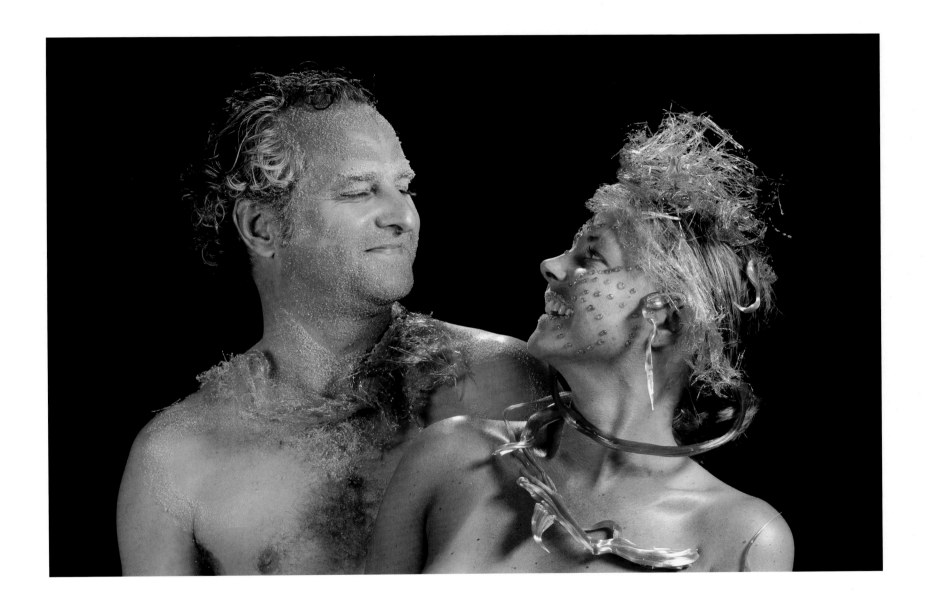

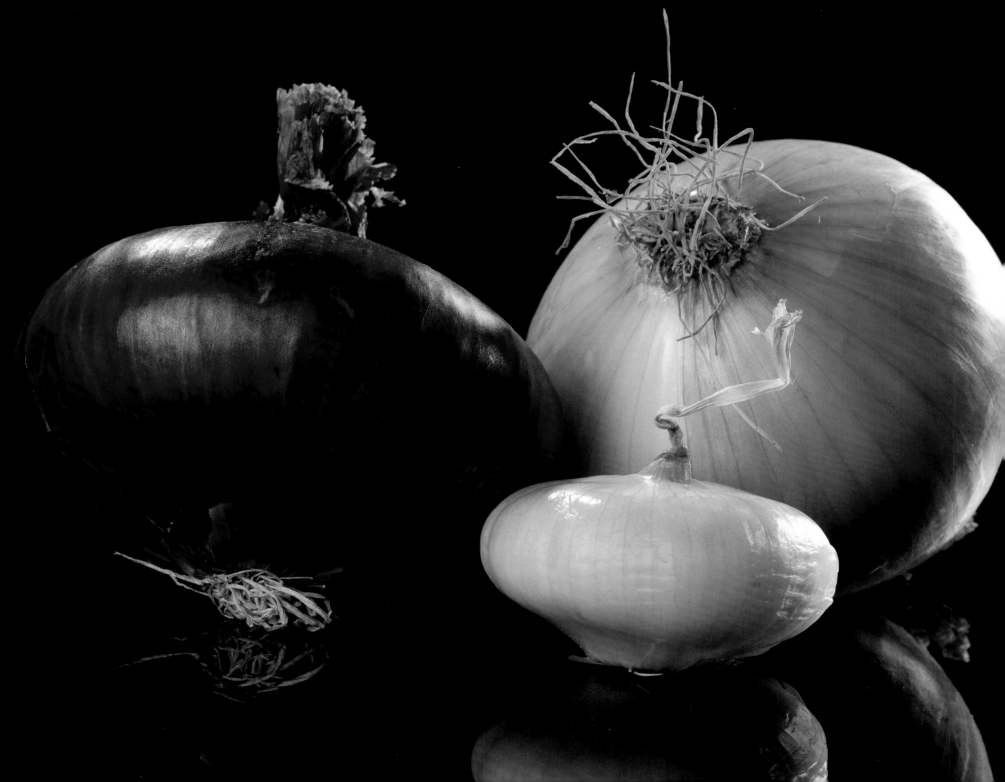

ONIONS

I DON'T KNOW WHAT I WOULD DO WITHOUT ONIONS. I adore this ingredient in any form: raw, caramelized, grilled, baked—that's only the beginning of what we can do with good onions.

If you ask me what is the best way to cook an onion, I will say every way is the best, but here is one of my favorites.

GRILLED ONIONS

WALLA WALLA SWEETS are the perfect choice for this dish, although any sweet onions will work. Choose several onions of similar size.

Remove the skin and slice round onion rings that are 1/2-inch thick. Try to keep the whole circle intact because it will be much easier to grill, and it will retain the onion's moisture, with wonderfully juicy results.

Make sure the grill is clean and heated to approximately 425°F. (It's easier to clean a grill when it's hot; be sure to use a wire barbecue brush.)

Brush each onion ring with a tasty olive oil and place them all on the grill. Close the lid and allow the flames to make love to the rings. The grilling time will vary, depending on the grill, the heat, and the onion. Be sure to check them after 5 minutes by lifting one side of the onion. If they have strong black lines from the grill, they're ready to be turned. Remove them when lines appear on the second side.

When the onions are done, sprinkle them generously with sea salt and place them in a single layer on a tray. Let them cool completely, then drizzle some very good olive oil over them.

Your onions are now deliciously ready to share. Forget the utensils: use your fingers and feed them to a friend.

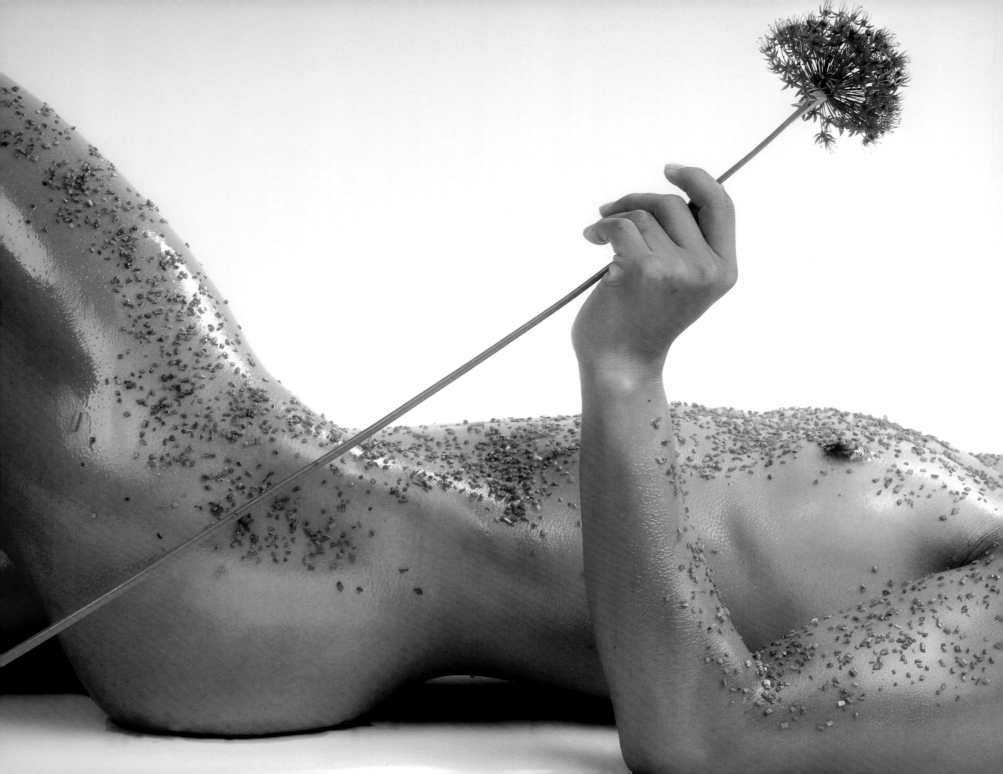

MAKING FOOD FOR A LOVER

HAVE YOU EVER MADE FOOD FOR A LOVER? Not for a loved one, but for a *lover*—someone you make love to. Cooking for a lover is a sweet expression of emotion not just toward that other person but for yourself too. Trust me when I say your efforts will be rewarded, no matter how the meal itself turns out.

I understand you might be intimidated by cooking, especially for someone you care about. Even if you think you can't boil water—it will be okay. Follow my suggestions and you will have a pleasurable and romantic experience neither of you will forget.

It is best if you make this evening a surprise. Do not promise to do it; just do it. That's my philosophy.

You've taken the first step, which is having the desire to cook for your lover and deciding you will do it. Now, you can enjoy the anticipation of using food to create a sensual evening. Look forward to sharing the meal and, more importantly, have no big expectations about any part of the evening. That way, you'll never be disappointed, and you'll be more open and receptive to whatever happens. (You never know—your lover might have a surprise for you too.)

Give yourself time—even a week—to plan the menu. Have fun while you think about the meal and the time you'll spend with your lover. Imagine the provocative ways you will show her your affection that evening. You should also ask about her favorite ingredients and her likes and dislikes. It is very important to ask if there is anything she won't or can't eat.

As the date night draws near, intrigue her by inviting her to dinner at your place. Request she wear something sensual. If she asks why, tell her it's a surprise. When the night arrives, make sure you are wearing something sexier than jeans—perhaps an apron that barely covers an intriguing part of your naked anatomy. Wear something that will enhance your creativity and release your inhibitions.

As you put the finishing touches on your menu, make sure the food items are designed to last all evening. Plan on serving drinks, two to four appetizers (four is preferable), the main course, and dessert.

I recommend your first appetizer be a frozen offering—something super simple, such as fresh frozen grapes, berries, or banana slices. Anything that will defrost in your mouth and taste delicious. Begin by feeding her with your fingers. Then add to the sensuality by passing the frozen food from your mouth to hers. Add a little zing by taking a sip of Prosecco—a dry, Italian, sparkling white wine—in your mouth before passing it.

For your second appetizer, choose something served at room temperature, such as figs and prosciutto. Feed them to her with your fingers and always remember to caress her lips. Pour a glass of rosé or red wine and enjoy it not only from the glass but from her luscious lips too. Let her do the same.

The third appetizer should be a cold one; I suggest oysters. Feed them to her from your hand as if it were the shell. Squeeze a small amount of lemon juice over the oyster before letting it glide into her mouth. Kiss her hand if she assists you.

Offer her more Prosecco, and this time, pour it into your hand rather than a glass. Challenge yourselves to dry your hand with your tongues. Remember, this night is all about sensuality and pleasure.

For the fourth appetizer, offer her something hot, such as fried zucchini blossoms stuffed with her favorite cheese, or prawns sautéed in their shells in order to make the most of their flavor. Peel the prawns for her, which is another way to share this delicious food and celebrate each other. As you feed her, caress her face with your hand and kiss her eyelids. Enjoy every flavor and texture of the food as well as each other.

I encourage you to keep the food simple. Remember, the less complicated you make it, the more time you will have to enjoy the experience.

Now it's time for dinner. Dinner in the United States usually calls for every part of the meal to be served on one plate. Well, let's change this for tonight. Instead, every dish should have its own plate, and the two of you should share it.

Are you hoping I will suggest a food item that serves as an aphrodisiac or that increases the libido? It's best if I do not tell you exactly what to cook for the dinner course. Trust me, in this situation, everything is an aphrodisiac because the main ingredients are the two of you: your touch, your taste, your smell, your bodies, your love.

The wine will help your efforts along too. Personally, I find good water very sexy, so even if you don't drink alcohol, the night can still be filled with romance. In this case, I suggest San Pellegrino or any naturally fresh juice.

Remember the cardinal rule: keep each course simple so you can offer more courses, because each one is an opportunity for kisses. Feeding each other with your fingers is erotic—and certainly easier than hassling with silverware.

Serve your salad last, after dinner, so it cleanses the palate and readies your taste buds for the fruit, dessert, and espresso to come. I recommend whole green leaves and dressing them simply with a little salt and a good olive oil. Don't add any vinegar: the extra tanginess you need for this salad will come from your skin as you use your bodies to feed each other.

Ahhh…dessert. The fresh mango or the chocolate? That is a tough decision. How about both but at different times?

If you start with the chocolate, blindfold your guest, offer her a sip of a good port wine, and then feed her a piece of high-quality chocolate from your mouth. If it's something creamy, like a mousse, simply use your finger.

By this point, I think your evening activities will be heating up and you will likely head to a different room...or you can always get creative in the kitchen, or on the couch or dining room table.

Don't forget the fresh mango and the espresso, although perhaps you will save them for the morning.

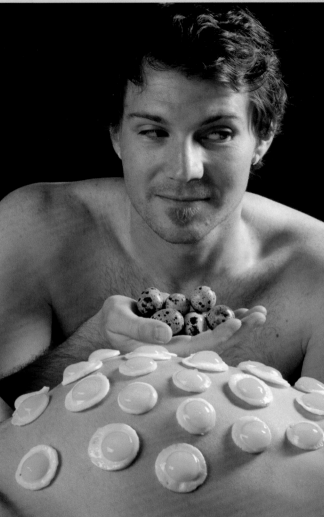

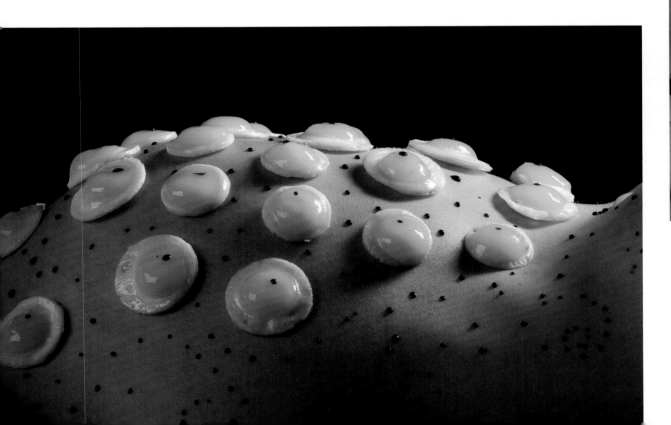

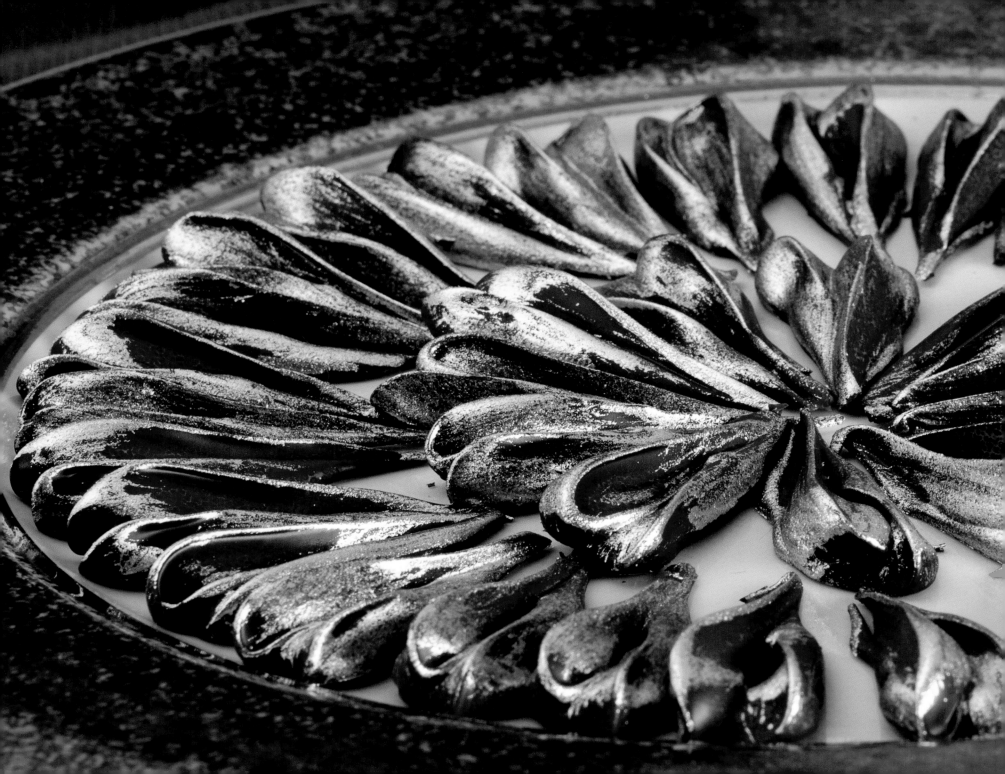

CHOCOLATE VULVA CALIENTE

CHOCOLATE VULVA CALIENTE is hard to find unless you know where to look but, I can assure you, it's worth the effort.

In 2005, I wanted to pay tribute to two of my favorite things by combining them: great chocolate and sexy women. Dark chocolate, I decided, was the best way to create and serve my own miniature version of a sensuous, touchable, lickable female body part—the vulva.

I added hints of lavender to my first set of little chocolate yummies because I've always felt this area on a woman's body is elegant, and I wanted a scent that would reflect this. I developed the recipe, lovingly made each one, served them to a huge, appreciative crowd at the Seattle Erotic Art Festival, and knew I was onto something.

About a year later, as I pondered another set of little dark vulvas on a tray in my kitchen, it struck me that not every woman tastes the same. Different women, different tastes. Maybe I should create different flavored vulvas as well.

The idea of actually translating the scents and tastes of various sexy women I knew into bite-sized chocolate vulvas I could share with other food-and-touch aficionados was exciting, so I set to work. After a lot of pleasurable research and several hilarious suggestions from friends, I developed a total of seven flavors for my chocolate vulvas: sea salt, citrus, rosemary, sage, almond, chili (caliente), and, of course, lavender. People go crazy for all the flavors, but the caliente—the chili-flavored chocolate—is the most popular.

The vulva can be a little too racy for some people, so I created a special chocolate heart to be served on a rose petal on Valentine's Day. I didn't use a chocolate mold—I did it freehand. With the technique I used, they came out looking like darling little butts. I call them my chocolate heart butts. People love these as well.

So, with my vulvas and my butts, I now have tasty and erotic treats that never fail to get people smiling and thinking and feeling.

I love feeding people. I love to be artistic. And, yes, I like to be provocative. Making chocolate vulvas and heart butts is a way that I can do all the things I love.

Go ahead and feed someone a special chocolate with a sip of good port or red wine and a kiss.

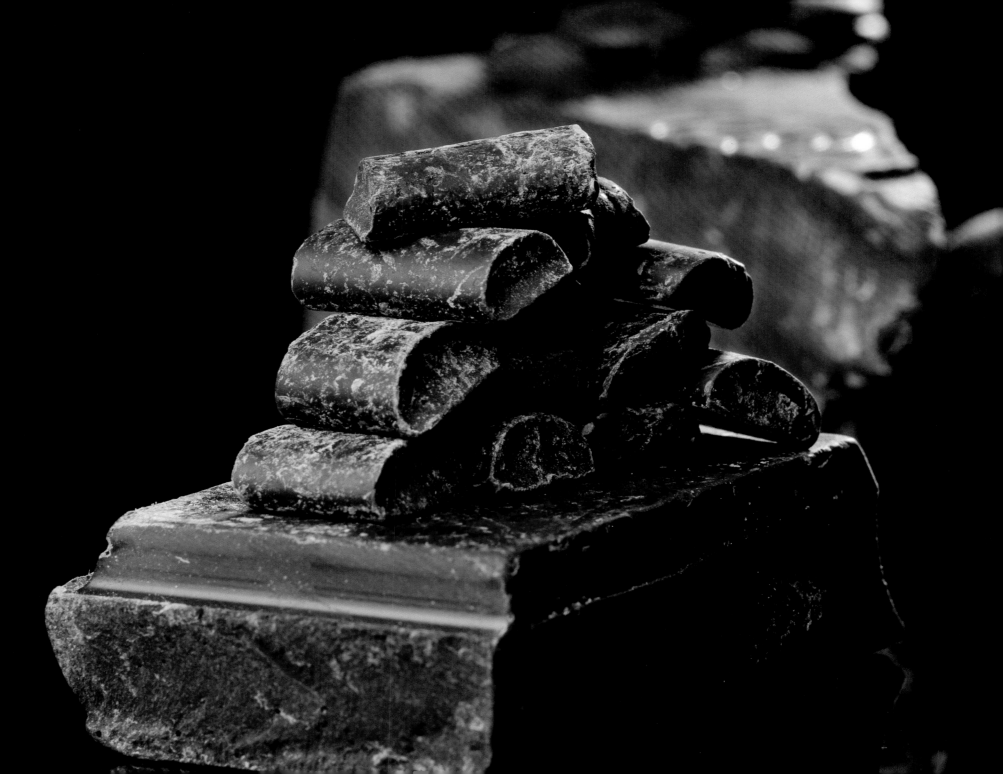

CHOCOLATE

WHEN IT COMES TO CHOCOLATE, I could write an entire book. A thick one. There are as many different uses for chocolate as there are people on earth. Like us, chocolate can be simple or sophisticated, strong or delicate, light or dark, prominent or subtle, warm or cold, soft or hard, traditional or innovative. Chocolate can also be a prelude or a postscript to making love.

Here are two simple recipes appropriate for a variety of situations, including your time spent alone, reflecting on the goodness in life.

TOASTED HAZELNUT CHOCOLATE BARS

Buy a minimum of 8 ozs. of good quality semisweet chocolate from the bulk section of your market. Chop the chocolate into small pieces, then melt them in a water bath over low heat. Make sure the water is simmering but not boiling or touching the bowl in which the chocolate is melting.

Once the pieces are completely melted, fold in 4 to 6 ozs. of toasted, skinless hazelnuts, either whole or broken into pieces. Pour the mixture onto a flat surface you've covered with clean parchment paper. Spread the chocolate to about 1/3-inch to 1/2-inch thick, and let it cool down completely. If the temperature in your kitchen is too warm, the chocolate will not cool properly, so place it in the refrigerator until it's slightly chilled.

When the chocolate is hard, simply break it into big chunks and eat some right away. Store the rest in a container with a lid in a cool location.

FAVORITE HOT CHOCOLATE

Super simple, super yummy warmth for your insides.

Chop 8 ozs. of semisweet or bittersweet chocolate into very small pieces. Separately, bring a cup of whole milk almost to a boil. Add the chocolate and whisk constantly until the chocolate is completely melted.

Pour into 4 small cups and serve it while it is still hot.

The next time you make this soothing and sultry beverage, add to the milk a small amount of orange zest or Grand Marnier for an orange flavor, or a splash of Frangelico for a hint of hazelnut, or a few drops of chili oil for a spicy flavor.

My mouth is watering. Is yours? I guarantee it will when you breathe in the steamy aroma of this hot chocolate.

Remember, with good chocolate you can seduce almost anybody. It works for me.

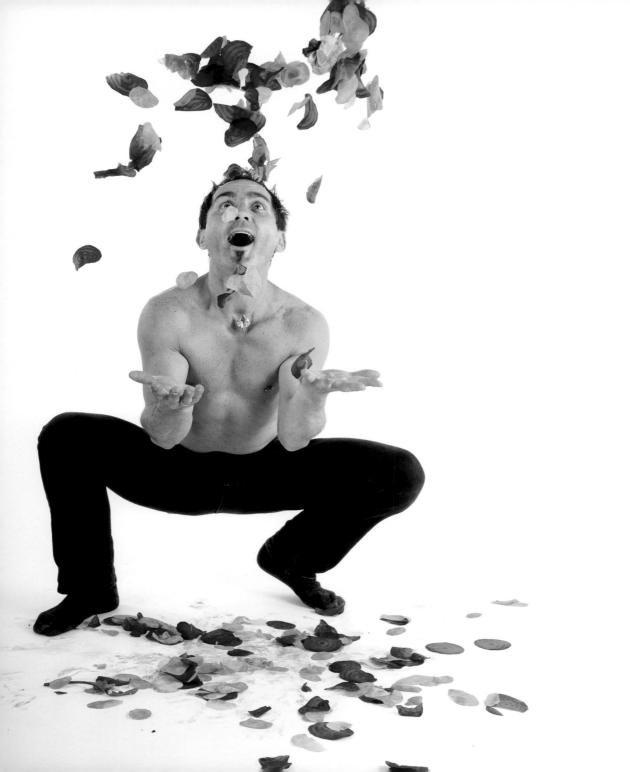

A PLEASURE ACTIVIST

I WENT TO THE 2004 SEATTLE EROTIC ART FESTIVAL wearing a black vinyl dress with a corset. And, if I do say so myself, I looked quite good. Throughout the evening, people told me how fabulous I looked. I never thought I was hot, but that night, I did feel handsome.

A man in a vinyl dress is certainly enough to command the spotlight, but I was also feeding people (by hand, of course) my signature candy for the evening: lavender chocolate vulvas. I had made each piece by hand, so while they all looked similar, each piece had its own little personality. I made about four thousand of them, and became so fast at it that by the time I had the chocolate tempered and ready to go, I could make three vulvas every five seconds.

That night was an incredible blast. The attention—okay, the *adoration*—I received was amazing but, at one point, it became overwhelming, even for an Italian like me. I escaped outside for a few moments to get some space and fresh air.

A pretty lady with her boyfriend came by and they asked if I could make some chocolates for a friend in California.

"Sure," I said.

"What do you do for a living?" she asked.

"I am a chef and an ethical slut."

"So you are a pleasure activist," she said.

"How so?"

"Because you like to give pleasure and because you like to feed people," she explained.

I nodded and we chatted a little longer before they continued on their way, but the conversation stayed on my mind. Pleasure activist? Hmm.

A couple days later, I was hanging out with my friend Allison and we were discussing what gives us pleasure. She observed that I am most happy when I am giving, cooking, or making love—when I share my message of loving people and loving life. She also said I am a pleasure activist.

It's a great title, I decided, after I'd had time to think about it. Pleasure activist was an appropriate description of my lifestyle.

A little later I relayed my new title to my friend Vanya (one of the models in this book).

He had a great laugh and said, "Here is one more for you. This is your new motto, Tiberio: 'I love everybody and you are next.'"

Yes! That is me. I do love giving pleasure. This is my trade, my craft, my skill. I am so fortunate to be who I am at this point in my life.

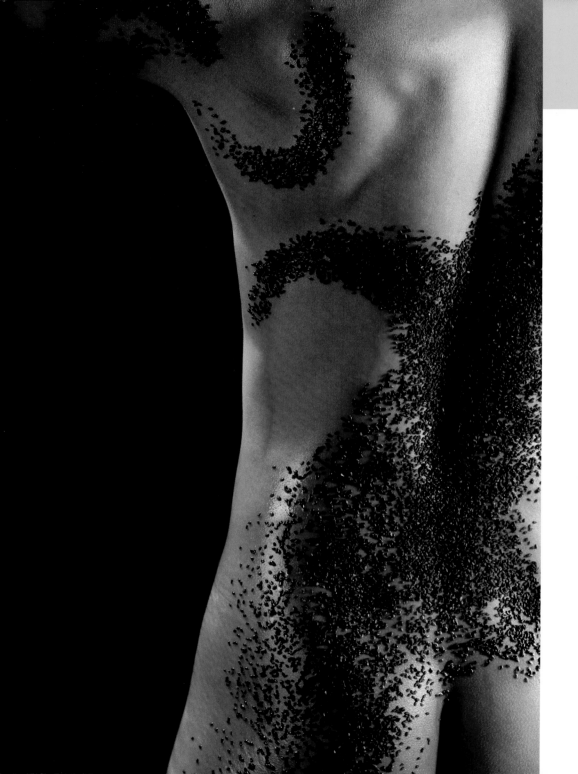

I am a feeder—of food, of pleasure, of touch—and a bit of a showman too, which gives me joy and attention. I love attention but only when I'm in control. You've probably figured out by now that I am still quite shy, deep inside, so I work hard to be more outgoing and to let my natural self shine through.

I raise my glass and say *Salute!* to black vinyl dresses.

(Guys, if you ever find the courage to learn to wear a dress—like women have learned to wear pants—I guarantee you will have a better chance of getting laid. Trust me, it works.)

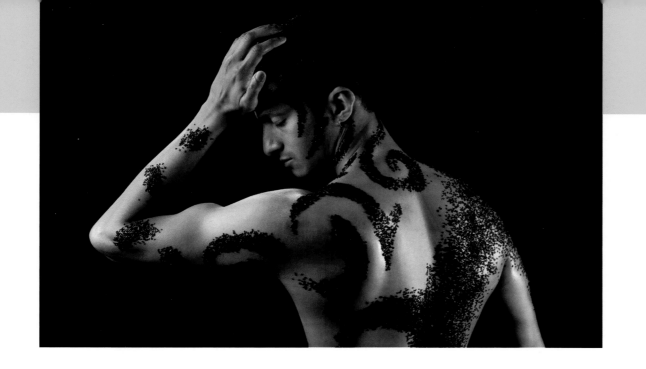

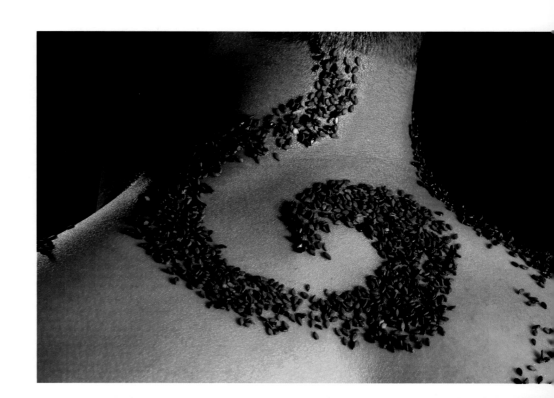

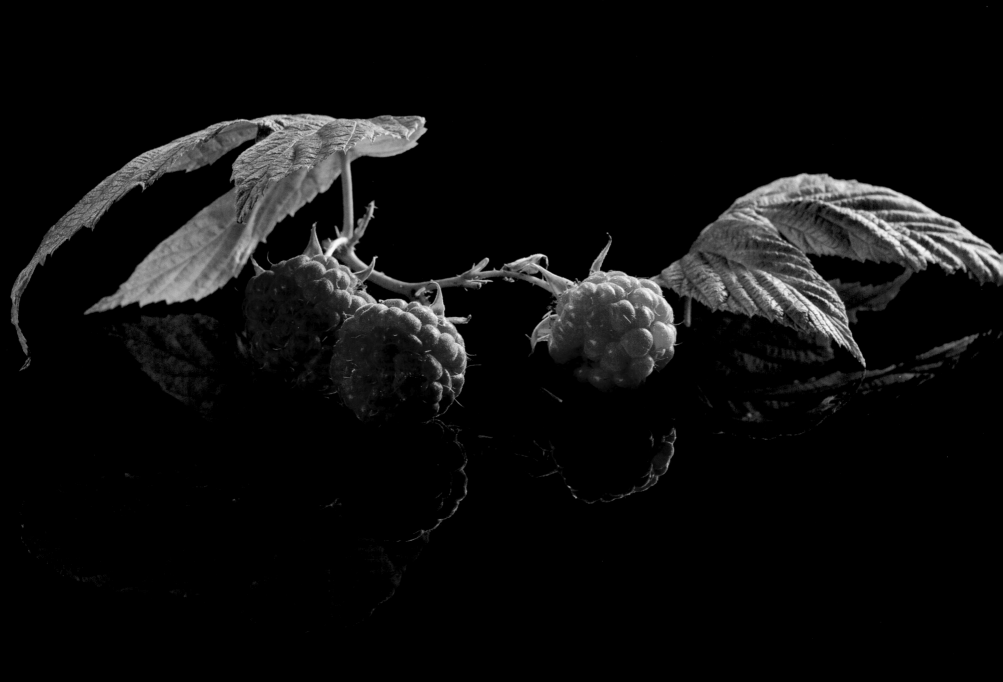

RASPBERRIES

A good raspberry needs only two fingers and a mouth. But if you are part of a couple and would like a playful and seductive activity, here are two creative techniques for enjoying raspberries—and each other.

RASPBERRY NECKLACE {

Begin with 2 cups of organic raspberries. Always make sure the berries themselves are firm, plump, and sweet.

Use a sewing needle, and fine fishing line as thread. Cut whatever length you think will work best for your neck, keeping in mind you'll need a few extra inches to tie the necklace. Gently push the needle through each berry, from the hollow end to the tip. Handle the berries carefully because they can tear easily. Thread the berries so they are spooning together—so they're cozy and beautiful to behold.

Once the necklace is complete, place it around your lover's neck. Instead of using your fingers to pluck and share a raspberry, use your lips or another body part—it's more fun and sensual as you enjoy the sweetness and texture of each delicate berry. The closer you keep the necklace to your lover's neck, the more that person will feel the heat or the tickling of your lips.

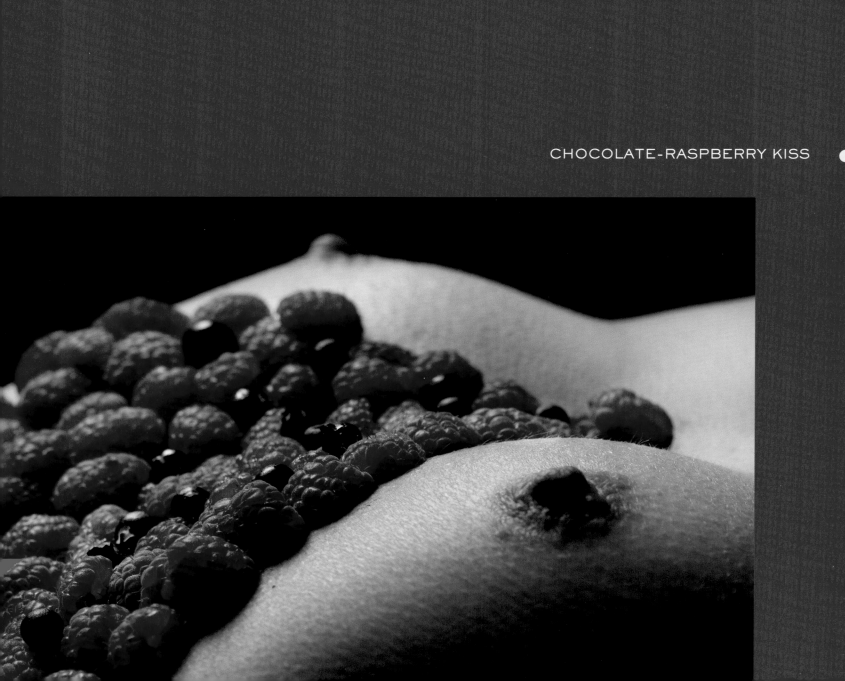

CHOCOLATE-RASPBERRY KISS

Buy or pick several cups of large, firm raspberries.

Using a double boiler, melt 4 to 6 ozs. of chopped semisweet chocolate. Be sure to melt it gently: do not allow the water to boil. Use a zester or very fine cheese grater to gather about 1 to 2 teaspoons of the zest of an orange. Avoid the white rind, as that part of the orange is very bitter. Add the zest to the melted chocolate and fold gently.

Form a cone with parchment cooking paper. Spoon in the chocolate and close the back of the cone. Cut the tip off and carefully fill each raspberry nipple. Place them in a bowl or tray in the refrigerator so they cool completely. Eat them all at once or at your leisure.

To add a creative twist, dip one side of one berry in melted chocolate and "glue" it to another berry, as if they are giving each other a succulent kiss. The chocolate will harden as it cools in your refrigerator, and your raspberries' juicy embrace will last longer. This creation works best if you plan to feed or seduce someone with your mouth. Since the berries are relatively small, it is difficult to share a single one between two mouths—two will do the job nicely.

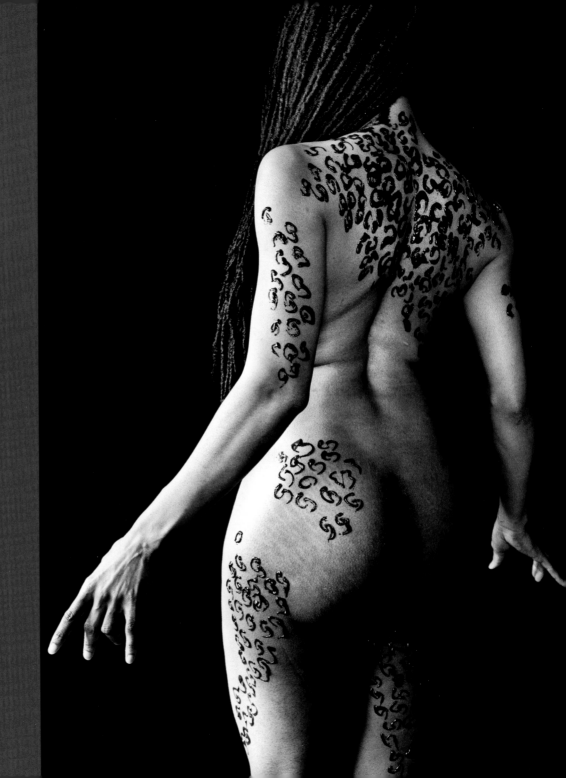

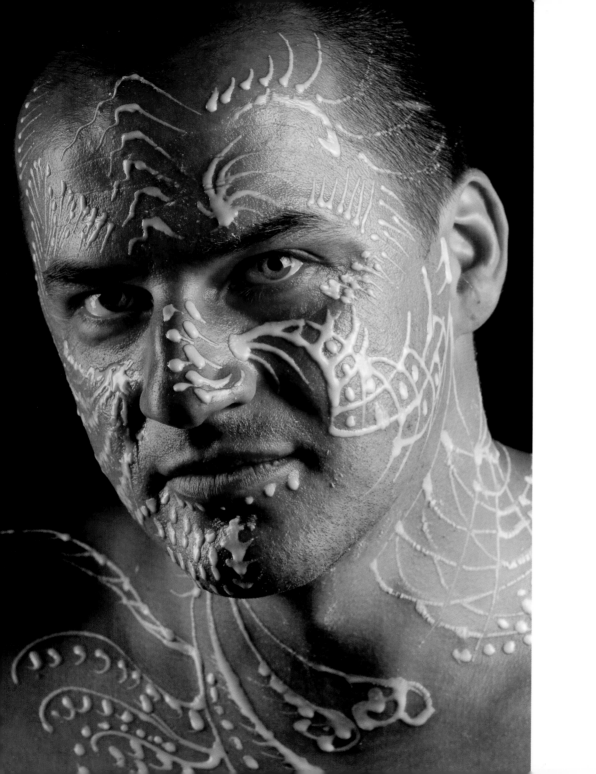

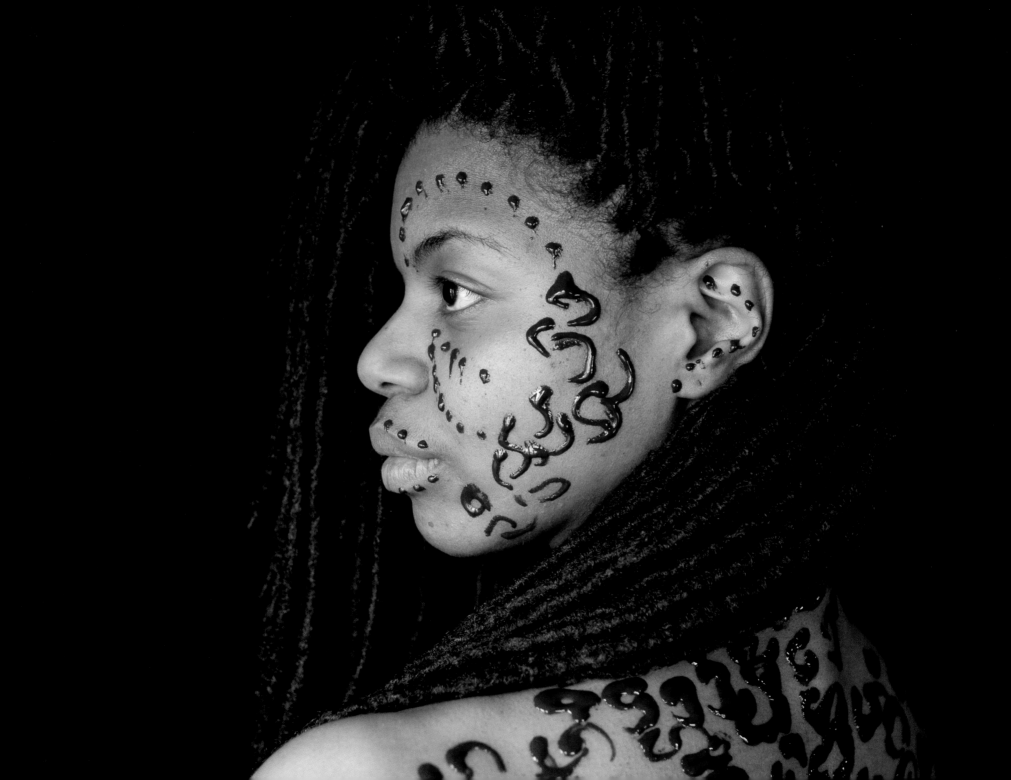

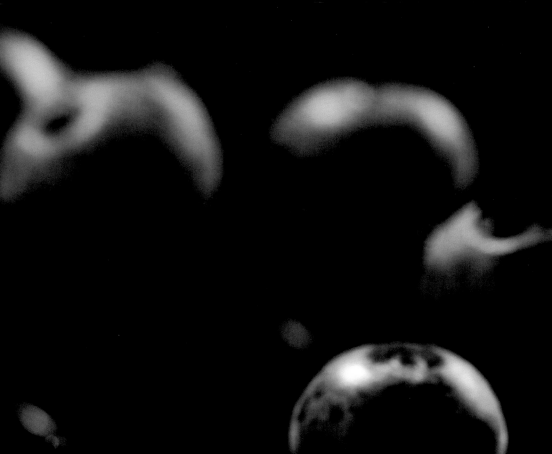

BLUEBERRIES

WHEN A LOVER AND I decided to take our relationship in a different direction and just be good friends, we parted in the most delicious manner.

She had previously asked me if anyone ever cooked for me, since I am always the one to cook for friends and for her. When she discovered that only my mother in Southern Italy does, she insisted on cooking for me on our final evening together.

She loved to use wild blueberries in her recipes and decided to include them in each course.

The menu she developed for our farewell dinner:

Crèpes with raw blueberries and melted brie cheese

Thin, pan-seared beef tenderloin medallions, served rare, with blueberry thyme and Barolo wine sauce

Arugula and fennel salad with blueberry dressing, shaved monchego cheese, and candied spiced black walnuts

And for dessert…

BLUEBERRY EVENING SEDUCTION

Starting with 1 pint of sweet blueberries, she folded in 4 tablespoons of honey and a teaspoon of freshly grated, superfine lemon zest. In a separate bowl, she folded 2 tablespoons of powdered sugar and a few seeds of crushed coriander into 1 cup of whole ricotta with 1 oz. of shaved semisweet dark chocolate. She scooped the ricotta mixture into an elegant dish, then topped it with the blueberries and a sprinkle of sea salt. She garnished it with a pretty mint leaf and served it with savory lemon crackers.

It was such a blessing of flavors that I felt happy, cared for, and appreciated. We made love for one last time.

That's what I call a happy ending!

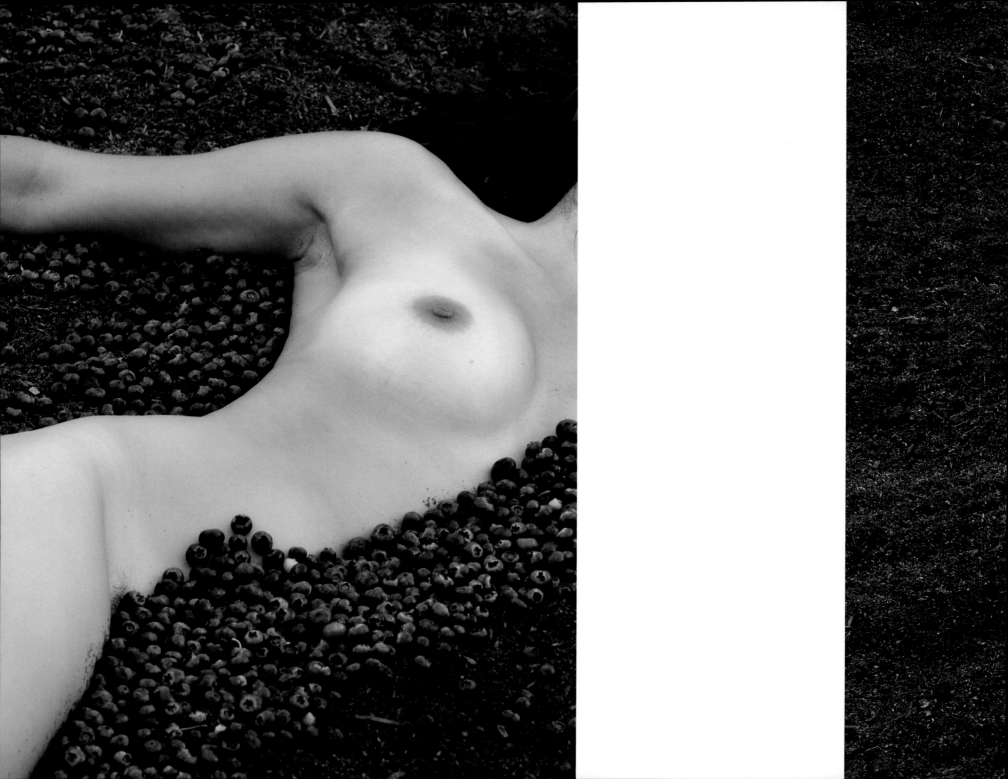

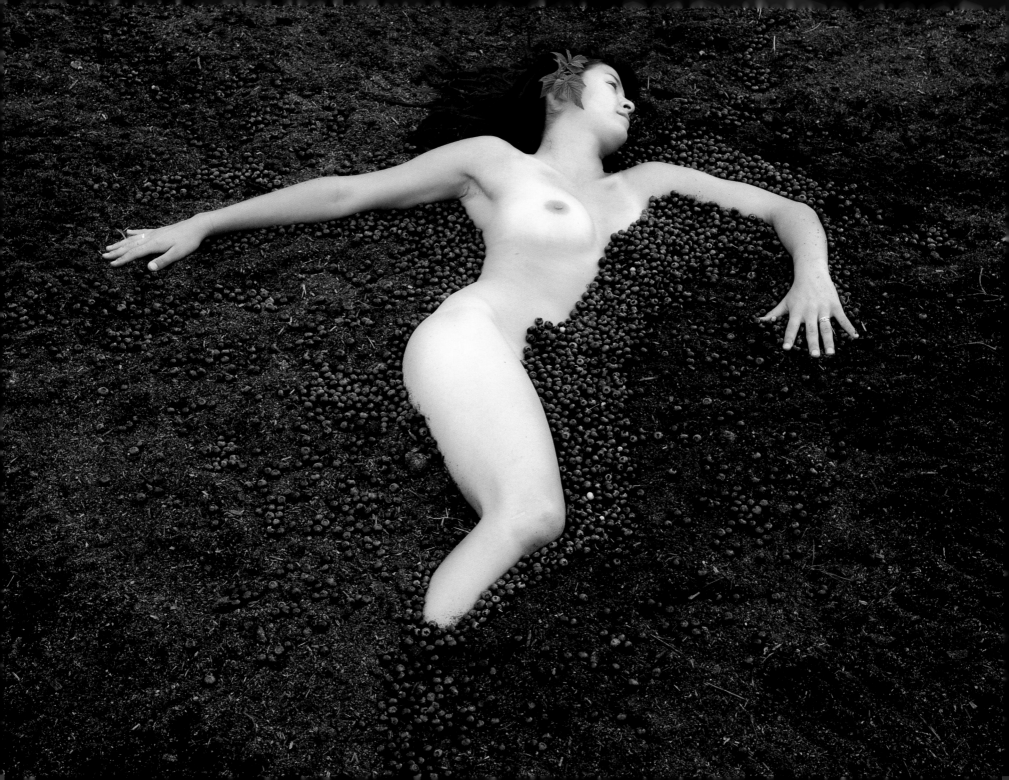

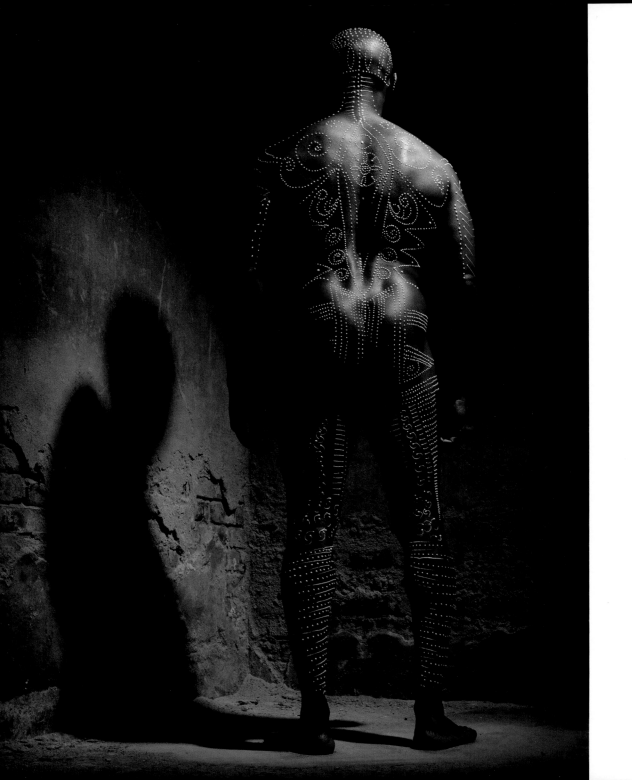

THE FACT IS WE CANNOT GIVE EACH OTHER
EVERYTHING WE NEED. SOME THINGS WE
NEED TO FIND ON OUR OWN; SOME THINGS
ONLY OTHER PEOPLE OR SITUATIONS CAN
PROVIDE.

CRAVING MAKES IT TASTE BETTER

DID YOU KNOW that if you eat lobster every day, after a while it will cease to taste like lobster as you know it? It will have lost the amazing flavor you craved. Your over-indulgence will have ruined its taste for you.

Without variety, or a little bit of time or space between feasts, even the best things in life can become mundane, bland, and less pleasurable.

The same is true for relationships that are not handled with a dash of moderation.

Compare my lobster example to a relationship with a new lover: The two of you can't get enough of each other. You want to spend every moment together. You crave the other person. It feels like the sex is non-stop, or at least it could be if only you could spend more time together.

So you do. You indulge yourself, and you partake of your new lover's delights. Or, in the case of the lobster, you sup on it every day. The lover/lobster relationship is exciting and you feel like it will last forever—nothing could possibly top this.

Things eventually change, of course. A few lucky people will be able to keep it up—the sex, the excitement, the intensity—but for most people, the novelty wears off and the brilliance dims.

The sex slows down. You might get back in touch with those old friends you pushed aside while you enjoyed your new lover. As the passion fades and monotony sets in, the sex may even become uninspiring. Your mouth-watering lobster now tastes…blah.

How can you avoid this common hazard? I think the idea of craving is the answer. It's the solution, not the problem. You don't need to satisfy all your cravings. Instead, you should recognize and applaud and enjoy them. If you give in to all your cravings all the time, where is the pleasure and the desire? If you eat lobster every day, you'll forget why you loved lobster in the first place.

Creating a little space in your relationship will help keep that anticipation alive. I suggest taking an extended break from each other at least once or twice a year: go on separate vacations, take a job that requires occasional travel, spend more time with friends, or use your free time to pursue one of your passions. These conscious choices will help you create the space every couple needs—even when they don't realize it. The fact is we cannot give each other everything we need. Some things we need to find on our own; some things only other people or situations can provide. I certainly don't mean you should change lovers as soon as the two of you have tried every sexual position in your combined repertoires,

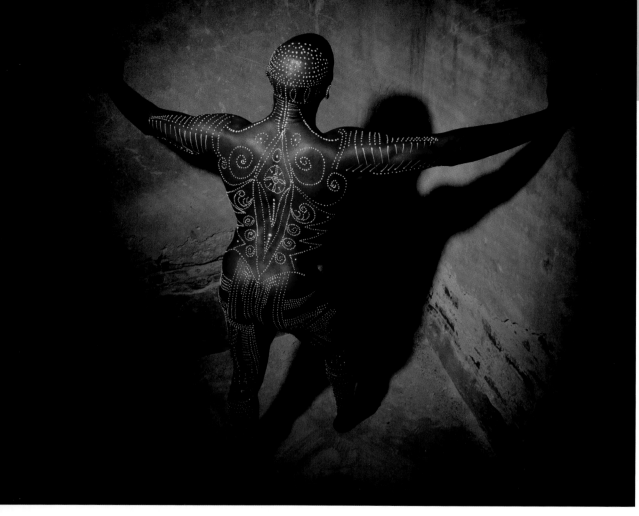

her. The sex is better, and we have more to talk about. The time apart is a good way to learn trust, to reflect on what we each need, and then how to communicate those needs in loving, respectful ways.

I give similar advice when it comes to food. Some people eat the same thing every day—day after day, week after week, and year after year. Are these people getting any real pleasure from that food? (Aside from the fact that they're not getting all the nutrients that eating a variety of food can provide.) The majority of people get sick and tired of the same thing, and they often don't even realize what a rut they are in. Eating lobster every day is not healthy; it means they're not eating other things that would undoubtedly provide different nutrients, and their spirits sag because their food and, by extension, their lives are monotonous.

I encourage people to go down a different path: try something new every day, adopt a different way of eating (become a vegetarian for a week, for example), or simply add a few proteins they haven't tried before. This way, the body and its taste buds will reawaken and feel invigorated—and hopefully bring nutrients to the body that had previously been lacking. So skip the lobster, and try instead another seafood item or something totally different.

nor do I advocate looking to someone else for excitement or intimacy if you're in a monogamous relationship. My point is that nobody is perfect, and even if someone was, perfection eventually becomes boring. Lobster ceases to taste like lobster.

Whenever I create a small space or some time apart in a relationship, I feel reinvigorated. I begin to crave my lover and all those beautiful things that had ceased to feel so wonderful when we were together too much. I'm eager once again to see

Later, add back in some of your old favorites—your lobster—but only occasionally. Now that you genuinely crave that food again, all that joy, anticipation, and desire will fill you up and satisfy all your senses, just like seeing your lover again after a little absence. Honestly, when you get ready to take that first bite of food, your mouth will water. When that old familiar flavor caresses your tongue, you'll be surprised by the intensity of the pleasure you feel.

Food and lovers are very much alike, aren't they? Remember to create space and allow cravings to intensify your experience. Your lovers and your food will remain appealing and exciting, and you will be the beneficiary.

Crave eating well, and *crave* making love.

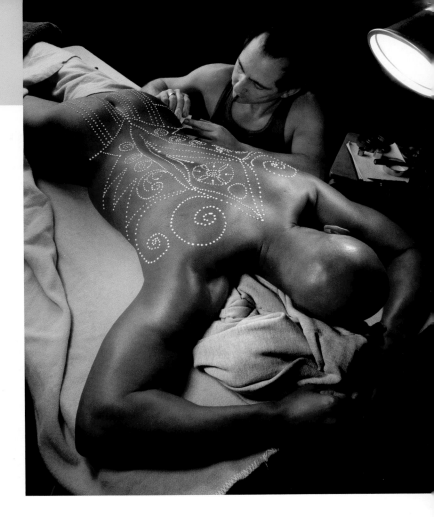

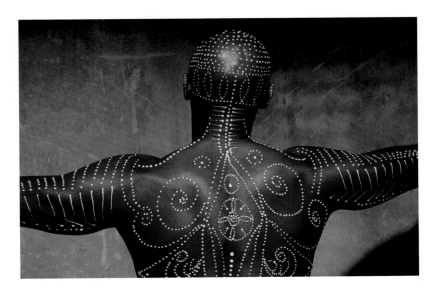

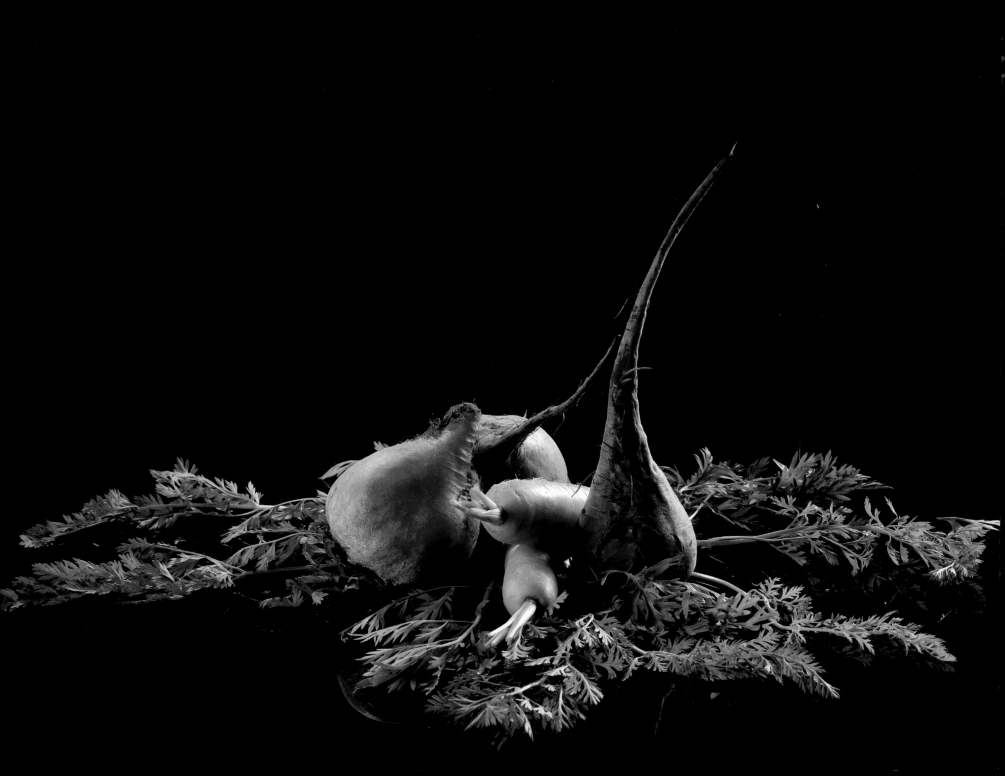

ROOT VEGETABLES

ROUND AND SMOOTH, firm and phallic, or curvy and cleft—I love root vegetables' distinctive shapes. When I see an array of them at a market or even nestled together in a bowl on my kitchen table, they remind me of a person's butt, legs, breasts, and thighs. Together, they make a beautiful body.

A few years ago, I made this delicious recipe, and it later inspired me to cover the bodies of a beautiful couple with these vividly colored vegetables. The models' paler skin was the perfect canvas for this particular food art. Now one of my favorites, this recipe's rich colors nourish and warm our souls from the outside, while the earthy flavors and nutrients replenish our passion and fuel our bodies from the inside.

ROASTED ROOT VEGETABLES

Gather about 2 lbs. of all the vegetables you love that come from under the ground. Consider using golden beets, red beets, turnips, carrots, daikon, parsnips, and any variety of potato you enjoy—sweet or purple or fingerling or even Yukon Gold. Be creative and uninhibited in your choices.

Preheat the oven to 425°F. When baked at a high temperature, these vegetables taste sweeter.

Peel the root vegetables and cut them into 1/2-inch cubes. To ensure even cooking, cut them all about the same size. Place them in a large bowl and add chopped garlic—at least 8 cloves or as many more as you'd like. Add 2 tablespoons of *fresh,* chopped rosemary, 2 teaspoons hot chili pepper, and sea salt to taste. Pour in enough olive oil to provide a good coating: about 1/2 cup.

After tossing all of the ingredients, take a small bite from one of the vegetables and suck on it for a moment. Let the flavor bathe the inside of your mouth. It's important that this recipe have enough seasoning, so use this taste test to decide if you should add more salt or garlic, or even some chili flakes if you prefer a hot and spicy flavor.

Arrange the vegetables in a single layer on a sheet pan or in a flat baking dish. Do not pile them on top of each other.

Bake your colorful and spice-freckled little root vegetables in the oven for approximately 20 to 30 minutes. To draw out the most intense flavors, do not remove them from the oven until every surface is crispy and brown.

This side dish goes well with almost any type of entree. I like to make extra because these vegetables are great as leftovers. Try eating them at room temperature too.

I always look forward to that moment when I remove these root vegetables from the oven. Their colors are so bright and beautiful—as if they've spent their entire lives primping for their big moment with you. That time is now, and they are so excited that they're bursting with color, flavor, texture, and aroma. I guarantee your tummy will love this great dish.

Buon Appetito!

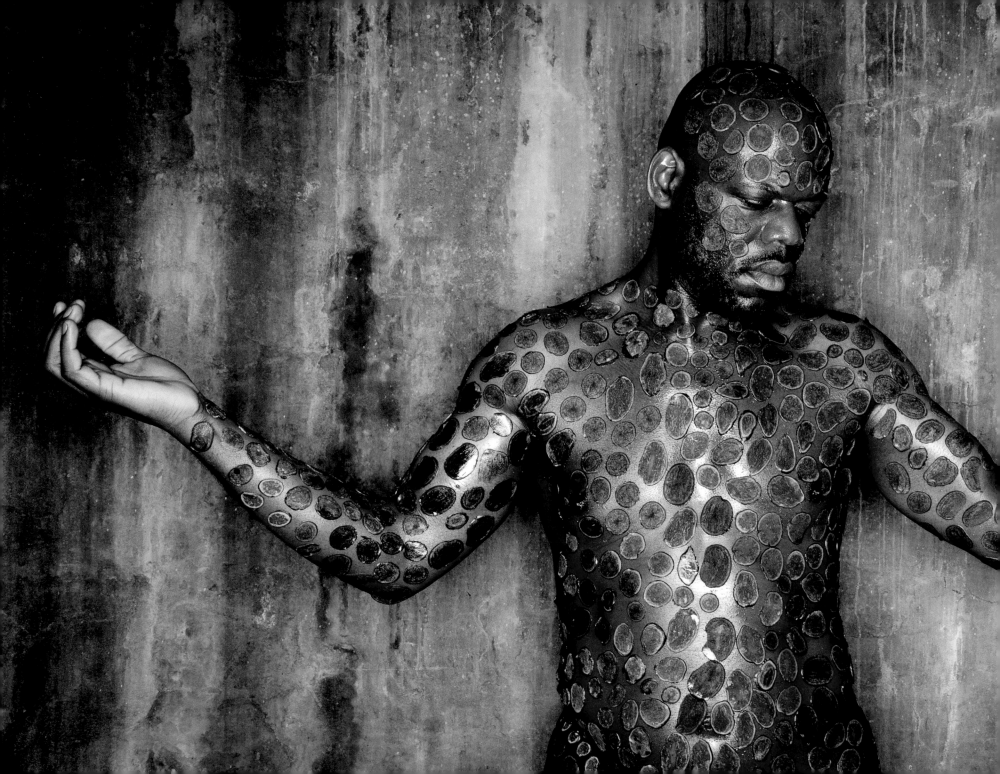

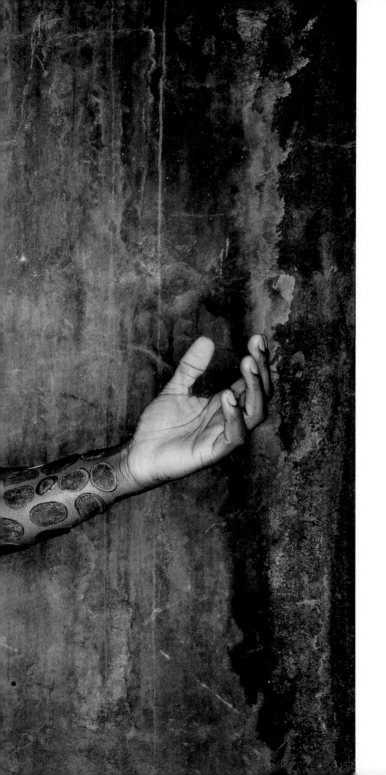
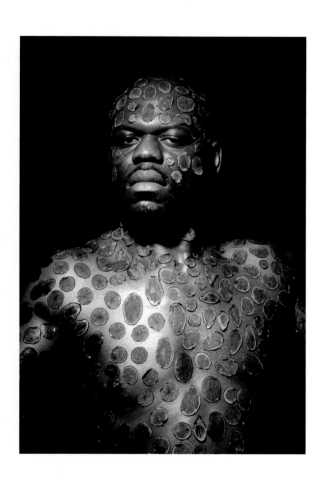

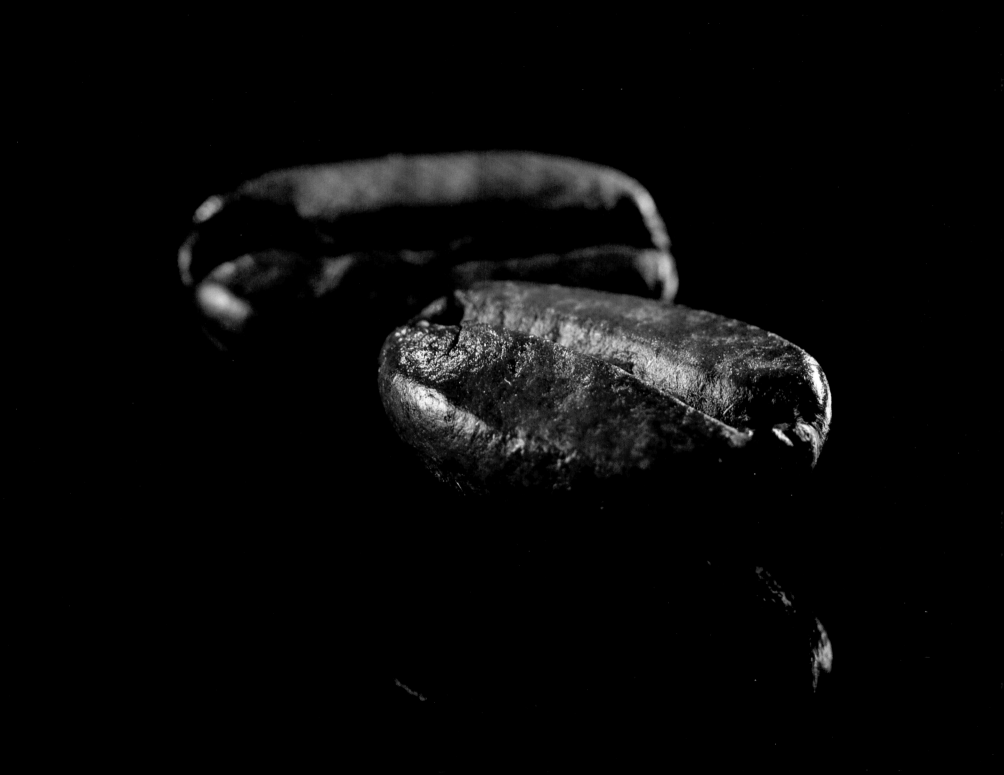

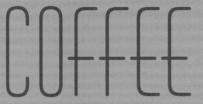

COFFEE

COFFEE IS IN MY BLOOD. In Italy, much like in America, we need coffee early in the day to revitalize our senses and restore our energy. Espresso is the morning drink of choice, and people flock to the bars to quickly down their first of several cups. An Italian bar is similar to an American coffee house—plenty of windows opening onto the street, a selection of baked goods, a friendly and relaxed atmosphere—but with the added benefits of elegant counters and colorful bottles of alcohol lining the back wall.

Drinking coffee is also a social activity suitable for any time of the day or evening. Relaxing at a bar or bistro in the neighborhood piazza, chatting with friends both old and new, leisurely sipping a hot cappuccino or espresso, watching the world stroll by—these are timeless, soul-nourishing moments.

My ultimate coffee experiences have come from a dessert my mother makes called *Dolce Mocha*, which is an amalgamation of biscotti, butter, toasted almonds, coffee liquor, and espresso. The recipe is secret, however, and I vowed a long time ago to never divulge it. Perhaps I will make it for you someday, and then you will understand the preciousness of this family recipe for the perfect coffee experience.

My mother's recipe is not the only heavenly coffee beverage I look forward to when I return to Southern Italy each year. On my first evening back in Neviano, I walk over to the local bar and order an Espresso Affogato, which is, literally, ice cream drowning in coffee.

ESPRESSO AFFOGATO

This is a very simple treat to make for a guest or for yourself, especially in the late afternoon or evening of a hot day. Be sure to use a good brand of vanilla gelato or ice cream, and high-quality espresso.

Select a small and elegant bowl, a half-moon dish, or a ramekin to prepare and serve your Espresso Affogato. Place a scoop of gelato into the dish, and make sure the scoop is only slightly smaller than the interior of the bowl. Pour a hot, freshly made shot of espresso over the scoop, and…that's it!

The hot coffee will melt the gelato, which forms a creamy layer on top of the dark espresso. The contrasts of light and dark, hot and cold, are striking. Soon, the two will blend and create a warm, thick, creamy espresso drink.

Do the same with a friend as the two of you use a small spoon to feed each other this companionable blend of two contrasting elements becoming one.

Che buono.

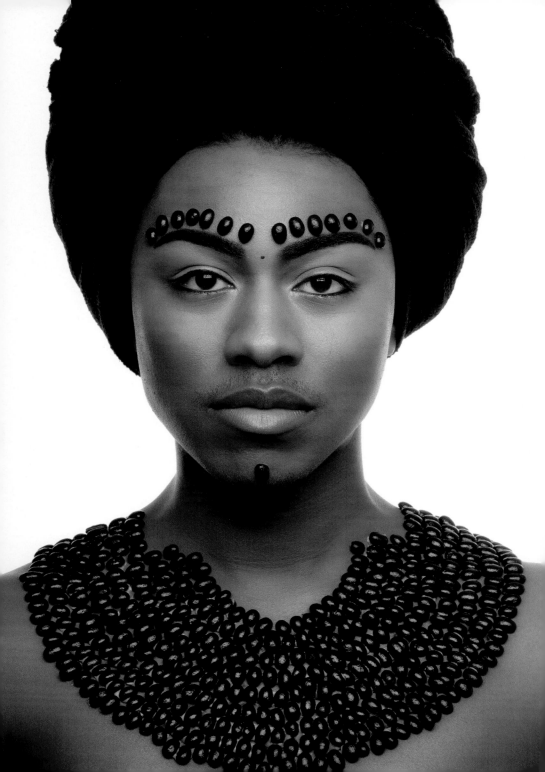

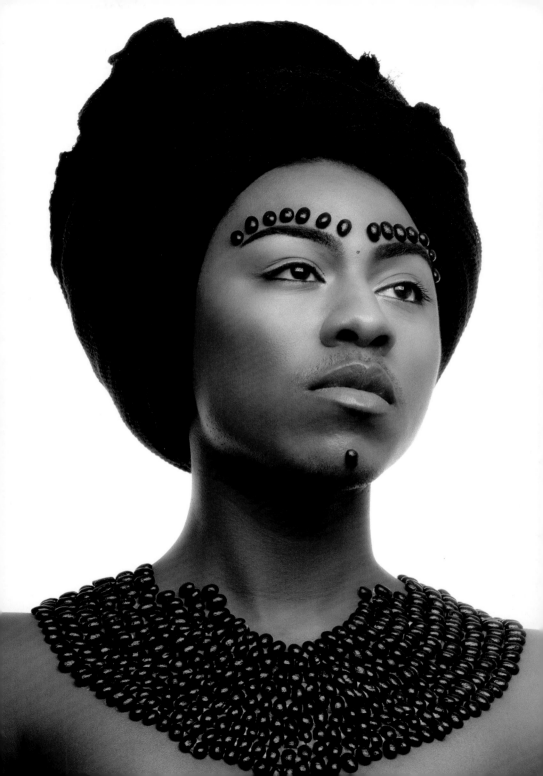

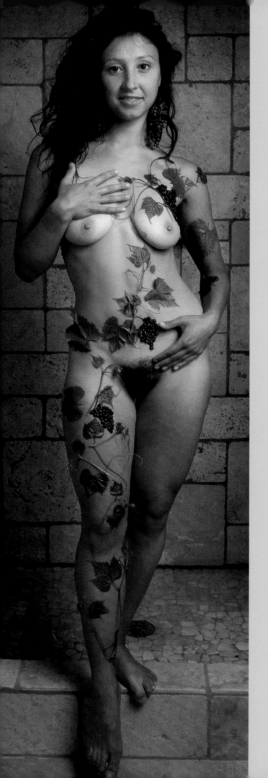

THE MODELS:
SHARING THEIR GIFTS

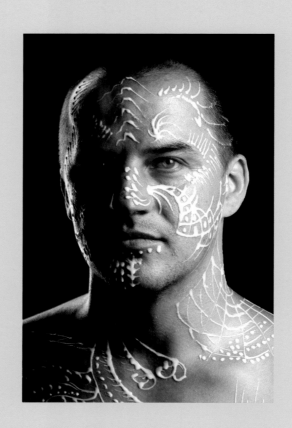

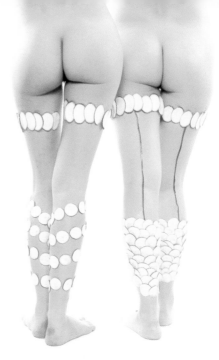

I LOVE THE MODELS IN THIS BOOK. Even though I worked with most of them just once, I still feel very close to them, as if they had been my models for a long time. There, I've said what I really feel: "*My* models!" We were meant for each other.

They are wonderful people, and I have been fortunate to work with them. Truly, the universe provided special people who have been generous with their bodies and spirits. Now, these are gifts all of us can enjoy.

Before this book was published, I used to show some of our photographs in a small photo album I carried with me. When people saw the photos, they frequently asked how I found and hired my models and how much I paid them. Everyone was surprised to find out that many of the models approached me about being in *La Figa*, and even those people whom I approached agreed to the photo shoots without any financial compensation.

In the beginning, I asked friends. Some immediately said yes, and a few declined because they weren't comfortable showing their bodies. With a couple others, I had to turn up the sales pitch, so I went in with the attitude of not taking no for an answer. This usually worked quite well, thank goodness.

After I started showing that small collection of photos, people eagerly volunteered to model. We had many requests and only limited time to do photo shoots, so we couldn't say yes to everyone. It was hard to turn down so many helpful, lovely people who were supportive of our project.

Even when we realized we wanted to use more people who don't look like traditional models, it was actually just as easy to find them. Once we started shooting those models, I purposely challenged myself to find new and inspiring ways to capture both the food and the body in a complimentary light. I'm thrilled, but not at all surprised, that their photographs are as joyous and enticing as the ones of our subjects who do look like traditional fashion models.

This decision to diversify the models certainly contributed to that building sense of pride and growing passion we felt.

One of the best things to come out of this project has been the relationship Matt and I have forged with the models. Each person is unique and contributed his or her own life story and experiences, which helped us create distinctive and memorable photographs. We are moved by the models' generosity. We're proud, too, of them and of ourselves.

More than anything else, however, we all had a great time, and now you get to enjoy and experience this collaboration with us.

COLLABORATING WITH MATT

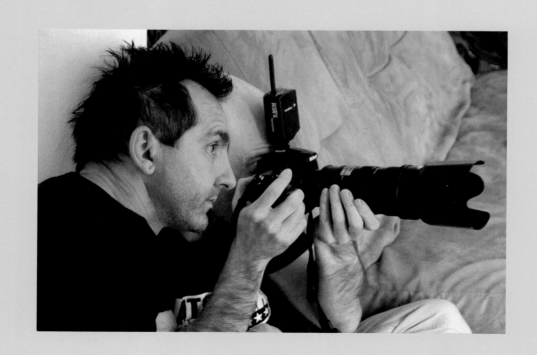

MY PARTNERSHIP ON THIS BOOK with Matt has been a great adventure, and I'm very fortunate to have been friends with him for the last ten years. We have learned to appreciate each other as artists who bring very different talents to the La Figa Project.

Matt and I had solidified our working relationship while building Saturnia, our art car for Burning Man 2002, but the foundations for *La Figa* really gelled in 2006, when we hiked in the Himalayas. We had done our first (and only, at that time) *La Figa* shoot a couple of months before we left for Nepal. During our trek, we talked about the possibility of creating an entire book of food and body photography. I told him we really needed to make it happen, and it would be fast and easy. Matt was interested in the idea, but told me it wouldn't be easy and would certainly take a year or two. Little did we know that the five-year journey of *La Figa* would make our trek in the Himalayas look like a stroll in the woods!

The twenty-five-day hike with Matt was a good testing ground to see how well we could work together under extraordinary circumstances. If our friendship could survive the ups and downs (both literal and figurative) of that unbelievably challenging journey, we could certainly collaborate on *La Figa*—and still be friends when it was done. Fortunately, we traveled very well together, and even when we got on each other's nerves, it was always easy to get back in sync. By the end of the trip, I knew Matt would be the official photographer and partner for *La Figa* (especially after I saw the incredible photographs he brought back from Nepal).

We wanted to start shooting as soon as we returned home, but we also had a lot of logistical questions that needed thought, discussion, and solutions. When I realized how complex this process would be, I was even more excited about the project because I recognized how unique *La Figa* would be. I didn't (and still don't) know of anyone else doing anything similar to *La Figa*—probably because few people would undertake the challenges that we were about to face. But we were ready for them.

Just as I'd hoped when I saw how well Matt and I worked together in the Himalayas, the challenges of *La Figa* strengthened our collaborative process instead of breaking it down. Over the last five years, we have jointly worked out many, many complications in our project and developed a rhythm that is spontaneous, creative, and fun for both of us and the models.

The partnership between Matt and me works for a variety of reasons. The key one is that we have great communication; we say exactly what's on our mind, and we are committed to understanding the other's vision. We are both professional, and we create a lot of good energy with the models. Matt is also very patient with my crazy ideas, and he does not get stressed out. Even though he is a phenomenal photographer, he does not have a big ego that gets in the way of the project. During the shoot, he takes countless photos, and he is open to taking the photos I suggest when I see something or a certain angle that I think may make a great image. He is receptive to my suggestions and will take my direction without being stubborn or resentful—but at the same time, he will let me know when what I want to do just does not make sense.

I spend a lot of time before the shoot making drawings of my concept. When I show him the sketches, Matt instinctively knows the best way to capture my vision as a photograph. At times I want to grab the camera and take pictures myself because I'm so excited to see those drawings come to life. Once or twice he has even handed the camera to me (no, none of those photos made it into the book).

Within a couple of days of the shoot, we get together to review the photos. There may be as many as 300 to 400 photos to sort through. Trying to pick the best ones is daunting. We each see the photos in a different way, and sometimes we do not understand why one of us likes a particular photo more than another. Matt sometimes does not grasp the importance of the tiny details about the food that I am so passionate about, and I sometimes don't get it when he insists that one photo is artistically stronger than another. Even though we each have our own vision and sensibility, we still reach an agreement. We somehow make it work—almost to perfection—and we're both extremely happy with the outcome.

Once we narrow it down to a handful of final shots, Matt works his magic on them. Though I always love the fresh-out-of-camera photos we select, when I see what he does with them on his computer, I am absolutely stunned. I am so happy that I want to kiss him. The combination of his artistic vision with his mastery of digital technology is what truly sets him apart from other photographers.

Working with Matt on *La Figa* has been an amazing adventure. I am already looking forward to our next project because I know that, whatever it is, it will be full of challenges and surprises and unexpected rewards, just like everything else we have done.

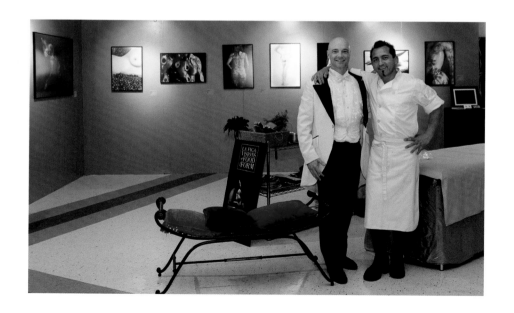

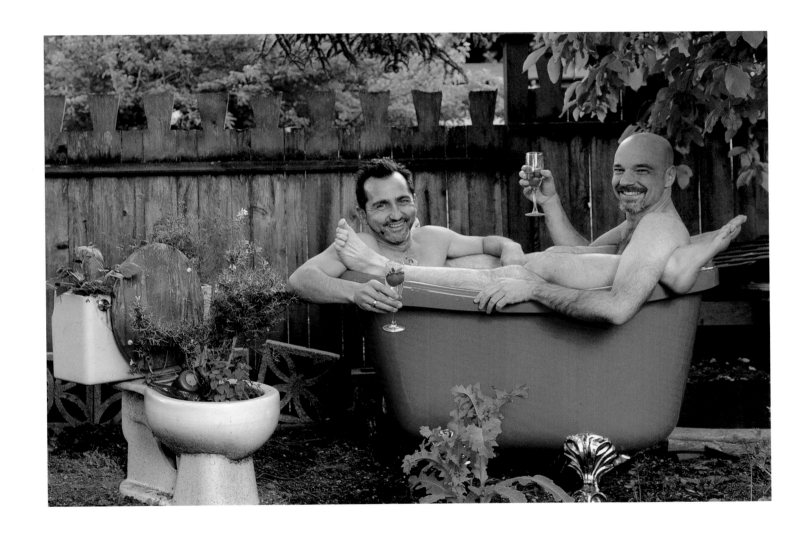

169

ABOUT THE PHOTOGRAPHY

BY MATT FREEDMAN

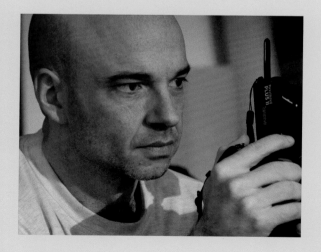

In 2006, when I first proposed to Tiberio that we do a studio shoot of the "food on nudes" performance art that he had been doing, I never dreamed it would grow into such an all-consuming and life-changing project. But more than fifty shoots and five years later, we are finally here—at the brink of having an actual book in our hands. The story of those shoots and that journey from there to here could make a book itself. But, instead, a few words about the photography will have to suffice.

Those who know me well enough may have noticed that my life has been composed of a series of nearly obsessive interests. One of my first was world travel. My overwhelming desire to share the amazing things I was seeing on my journeys was what led to my next obsession—photography (we will just skip over the obsessions with percussion, salsa dance, snowboarding, etc., for now). Travel photography is, of course, much more about finding images than creating them from scratch. When I am in my photography "zone," I see the world around me as a flow of two-dimensional still images, and I am constantly hunting for the truly amazing ones—both to remember what I was experiencing and to be able to share those experiences. My view of the world is actually more two dimensional than most people's—an extremely myopic left eye leaves me with rather poor depth perception. So perhaps I literally do have a photographic eye?

The style I have developed in all of my imagery is informed by these roots. Though carefully staged studio work may at first seem to be the complete opposite, the *La Figa* book project is actually travel photography for me. Every time Tiberio and I do one of our shoots, it is like a journey to a strange and exotic new world, with its mysteries unfolding before our eyes. Before the two of us trekked for a month in Nepal, I of course did deep research on it and looked at countless photographs (including my own, from ten years before). But still, I was completely surprised by the magical images I was able to bring back from that journey.

Similarly, we plan each of our *La Figa* shoots in great detail—Tiberio knows which ingredients he will be applying and what the design will be. We often work out a rough pose in a test session before we even go to my studio. I will decide in advance how I want to light the shot and which background will work best for it. Despite all of this advance planning and pre-visualization, I am always amazed at what I see as Tiberio creates his ephemeral art on the model's body. And even more amazed by the images I bring home.

When he has finished applying the ingredients, I get the same feeling I do when I walk out the door for a stroll in an unfamiliar foreign city—the hunt for images has begun. Like with travel photography, it is easy to get passable snapshots. And with a destination as strange and exotic as food on a naked body, it is not too difficult to get shots that are silly, ugly, unflattering to the model, or just plain weird. It is another matter entirely to create a photograph that is itself a work of art as powerful as what Tiberio has created in front of me. I know that there is a mind-blowing image in there somewhere—the challenge is hunting it down.

Our single biggest photographic challenge is the posing. For many of the shoots we have done, once the food starts going on, the model can not move. So we work hard on getting a pose really dialed in before Tiberio starts applying the ingredients. And standard textbook poses rarely work for these shoots (especially the shoots with more than one model), so we are constantly improvising and experimenting. Added to the mix is that, for the most elaborate designs, the model must hold the pose for two to three hours, so we have to find something that is extremely comfortable for him or her.

The lighting is the next most crucial element of each shot. Though we have done some location shots, I generally prefer to shoot in my studio, so that I have absolute control over the lighting, and a full arsenal of tools. I intuitively know what type of lighting arrangement will look best for a given pose and food arrangement, but I do a lot of experimenting and fine-tuning with the lights as Tiberio is applying the ingredient du jour. After that, it is a matter of finding the camera angle and the perspective (i.e., distance from the model combined with lens focal length) that brings the image together into a final composition that works.

As on any voyage, serendipity can sometimes play a huge role. For example, one of our favorite shots is the one of the woman with chocolate on her back (page 145). What makes that shot for me is the extreme tension in her body and hands. I did not visualize that, let alone direct her to tense up for the pose. In fact, Tiberio had just finished applying chocolate to her inner thighs—which were incredibly ticklish—and she was still laughing hysterically when I pressed the shutter, which is the tension that is captured in the image.

Of course the journey does not end when we leave the studio—the real exploration for me begins when I have downloaded the images to my computer. First, the (usually painful) process of deciding with Tiberio which shots—sometimes out of hundreds—are the keepers. Then, for those, gradually teasing out the full potential of each one. For a typical *La Figa* shoot, I will easily spend two to three times the amount of hours on the computer with the photos than we actually spent in the studio (and we spend *a lot* of time in the studio).

Some of the destinations we have reached in our *La Figa* shoots were easy, fun, and just plain delightful, while others have been incredibly challenging and stressful. But the most difficult journeys are often the most rewarding in the end. The images in this book represent my absolute favorite keepsakes from my fifty-plus journeys with Tiberio into the world of *La Figa*. I hope you enjoy them as much as I enjoyed the travels.

THE MAKING OF LA FIGA

THE ART AND THE COMPLICATIONS

WHEN I CAME UP WITH THE IDEA for this new art form, I had everything planned in my head and thought it would be relatively easy. What's so hard about putting food on a body? I'd been creating art with food as a pastry chef for the previous two decades; I knew food inside and out, literally, and I also knew the human body—especially the female form—just as well. Sure, it would take a lot of time to create the photographs, but I was motivated, and my visions of food and form inspired and sustained me.

Once Matt and I started shooting, we quickly discovered that I needed to figure out how to get the food to stay on the models' bodies when they were not lying down. And it had to be there for several hours, without moving or sliding, and still look as fresh as when I first placed it there. On top of that, I chose to use only edible ingredients in our photo shoots—and that included the various adhesives I would have to invent. As it turned out, some mixtures worked great with a particular food ingredient or on a certain skin type but didn't work well at all at the next photo shoot.

We quickly realized another of our biggest challenges was that, once the food was on the model, he or she could no longer move. At the beginning of the shoot, we had to place the model in the right position for the shot we needed, and it had to be a position he or she could hold for up to several hours. We worked as quickly as we could, but…Mamma mia! Our models have had the patience—and the bladders—of saints.

Matt and I have created a special relationship with the models over the years. We found the best way to have a successful photo shoot was to first start with a dinner at my home, in advance of the shoot date. We invited the models for a lovely dinner that I cooked. This created a relaxed atmosphere and gave us a chance to talk about what we wanted to achieve with the photo. After dinner, we tested the food I'd selected on their skin to make sure there was no adverse reaction to it. When we were satisfied with those tests, we worked on the pose so we had a rough idea of what we would do in the studio. This was a lot of fun and helped our models better understand what would happen on the day of their shoot.

During this project, I have learned things about food that I never did in my career as a chef. No one could have taught me these things—there was no "How To" manual. I needed to go through this experience myself. For example, to get ready for the first photo shoots, I spent many hours at my house, learning how to make food stick to a mannequin…which ultimately didn't help, because the mannequin was not made of warm human skin (though I still sometimes use her as I sketch designs). Grocery shopping was a little frustrating too, because sometimes I had to go to four or five places to find the perfect ingredients, only to arrive home and find they were already dried out, bruised, or simply looked dead.

Another complication I found—usually midway through a photo shoot, because this particular issue wasn't always apparent during our planning meetings—was the model's skin type. Some people had dry skin while others had skin that was quite moist. If the skin was dry, some types of vegetables and fruits did not last long because the skin sucked the water out of them. Then they dried out and looked terrible—unappealing, unattractive, lifeless. Or when there was sweat on the body and the food slid off—that was difficult to deal with, especially when a sticky ingredient that worked on one sweaty body didn't always work on another.

The color of the skin was also very important. Some food ingredients looked great on a person with a certain skin tone and terrible on someone else with a different one. When I worked with sliced food, it changed color, of course, after it had been exposed to the air and the warmth of the model's skin. I dipped the food slices in citrus water to preserve the color, but sometimes the water irritated the model's skin.

And what else did I learn? A hairy body will not work at all for these shoots. Food plus hair is never a good match.

To be honest, I have had more than a few moments of doubt during this project. I spent many nights without sleep; a couple times I almost got in a car accident while driving because I was consumed by planning a shoot, and my thoughts were not on the road. Even when I was teaching a cooking class, I could not stop thinking about what I was going to do with a model whose shoot we had scheduled.

On the days when I was overwhelmed with these challenges, I certainly felt like giving up. But I didn't. I am glad I hung in there and figured out new ways to solve problems. After all this work, I feel like I have finally mastered my art of food and form.

I appreciate and celebrate everyone who was involved in this project, especially Matt and all the models who loaned me their bodies and took this unconventional journey with me.

I knew it was important to follow my heart. I'm glad I did.

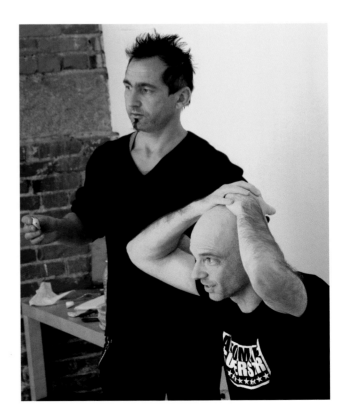

BORN IN NEVIANO, a small town in the "boot heel" of Southern Italy, chef-author and cultural provocateur Tiberio Simone is a James Beard Award-winning food artist.

Simone's formative memories of youth are of the traditional, homemade foods grown on the farm and prepared in his mother's rustic kitchen, such as home-baked bread with fresh tomato, olive oil, and basil.

After experiencing a string of vivid, personal upheavals in his early life, Simone ran away, trading the domestic violence at home for the more perilously mean streets of Southern Italy. At the tender age of eighteen, he enlisted in the Italian Armed Forces, where his quick thinking and street-wise demeanor served him well as an elite paratrooper.

Simone then met an American girl who became his wife and introduced him to another world in the United States. Thus began his culinary career at age twenty-one in an Italian restaurant in Seattle, Washington. He quickly recognized his passion for cooking and worked in kitchens across the city with many different chefs, mastering a wide range of cooking styles and techniques along the way. Simone was so enamored with the culinary arts that he took on a second job—unpaid for two years—learning the art of pastry. Subsequently, Simone was hired as pastry chef at the landmark Four Seasons Olympic Hotel. In 1995, he won the coveted James Beard Award for his creation, Hazelnut Decadence Crunch Cake, which critics described as an orgasmic amalgamation of nuts and chocolate.

Years later, tired of working as a chef for luxury hotels, Simone launched his own company, La Figa Catering. Becoming a small business owner allowed him the mobility and creative freedom to express his love of food and sensuality through a range of culinary arts. At the same time, Simone became involved in the worlds of performance art and theater, where he experimented with decorating the human form with food.

La Figa: Visions of Food and Form arose not only from the success of those performances and the passion for his art but also from his desire to share a vision of a life made full through a diet of both food and sensual touch.

For me, the sensuality of food closely resembles the pleasures of sex. From the first bite of a meal, the body is catapulted into rapture through the last climactic bite. A delicious morsel is as sweet as the first kiss.

—Tiberio Simone

LONG-TIME SEATTLE RESIDENT Matt Freedman is a professional photographer and professional technologist. From an early age, he was also an avid amateur film photographer. But not until digital technology matured at the turn of the twenty-first century did his involvement with photography truly emerge. Once he could manipulate the creative process on a computer, instead of in a darkroom, his interest quickly progressed from hobby to obsession.

Freedman's natural artistic vision, combined with his technical acumen, helped him master the art of the digital image. He was soon sharing his photography with a growing online following, exhibiting his work at venues such as the Seattle Erotic Art Festival, and publishing his work in the books *Trekking Nepal: A Traveler's Guide* and *Artivisme: Art, Action Politique et Résistance Culturelle*.

In 2007, Freedman merged his skills in photography and technology to become the staff photographer and director of technology for *JUST CAUSE*, a bi-monthly magazine about individuals, organizations, and businesses "doing good" in the world.

Freedman went on to produce *Burning Man 2008: A Photo Essay*, which was the first iPhone app about the Burning Man festival. Described as a "coffee table book for the iPhone," the app is a product of Freedman's photography, writing, and software engineering skills. An excerpt from the app is now the official guide to photography on the event website, making Freedman perhaps the world's leading expert on Burning Man photography. He is also the author of mRelease, the first iPhone app for photographers to create model releases in the field.

Although primarily self-taught, Freedman also studied at Photo Center Northwest in Seattle. During a Form and Figure course in 2006, Freedman asked long-time friend Tiberio Simone to work with him on the final project. That first photo shoot began a lasting collaboration which—fifty-plus sessions later—produced the book *La Figa: Visions of Food and Form*.

The style I have developed in all of my work could be described as journalistic. Whether exploring a foreign country or doing an erotic studio shoot, I do not take images so much as seek them.

—Matt Freedman

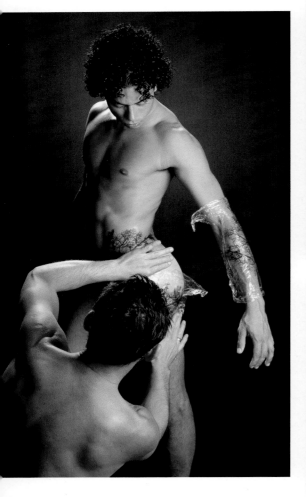

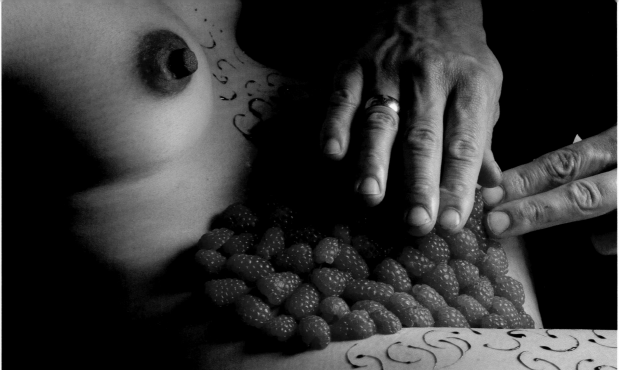

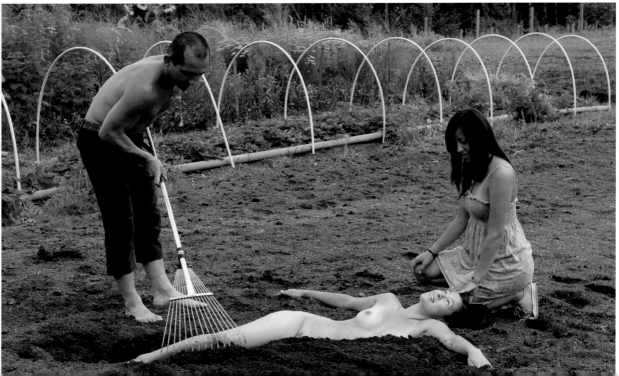

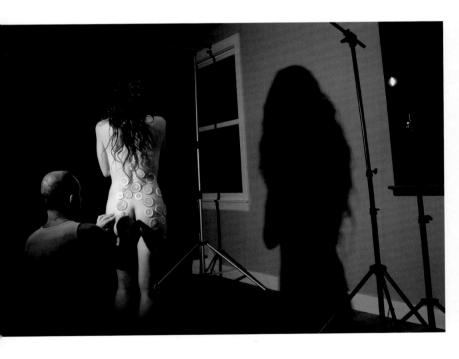

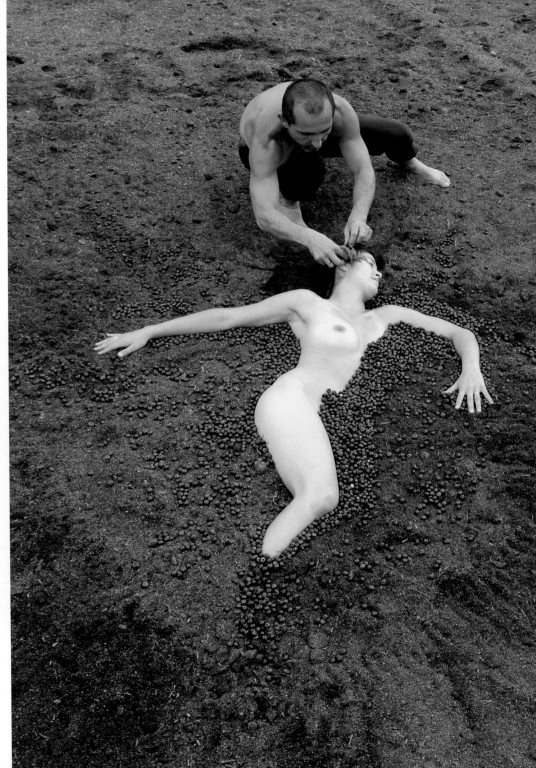

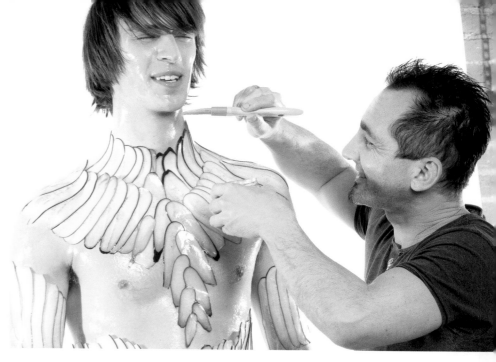

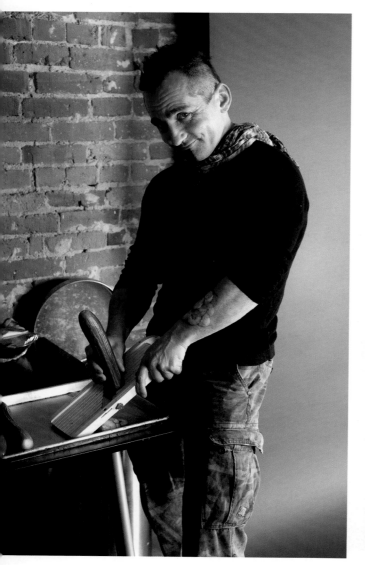

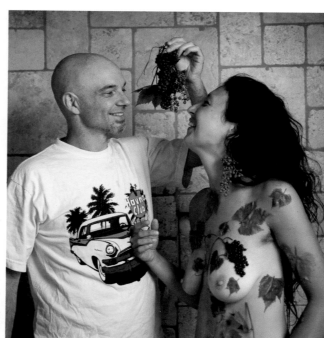

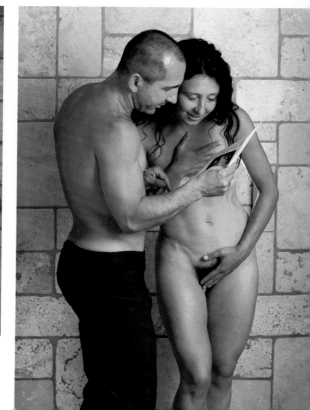

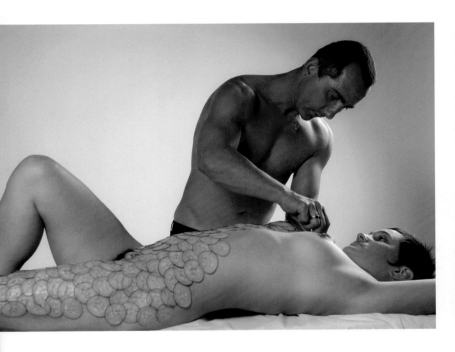

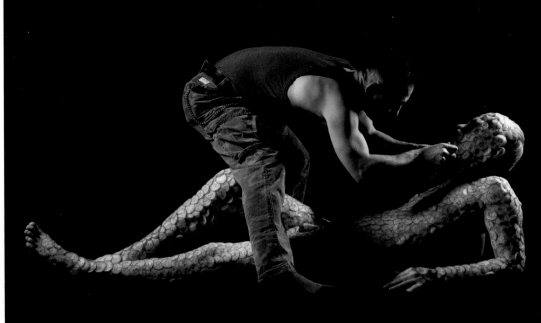

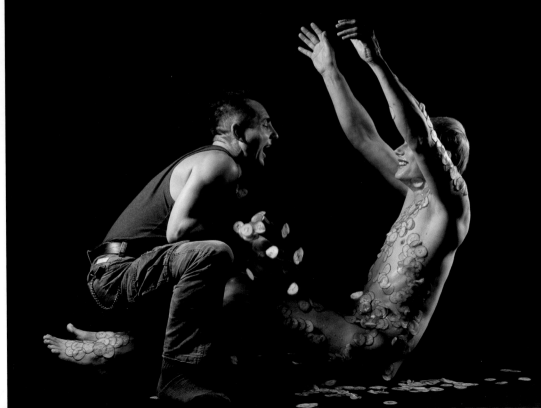

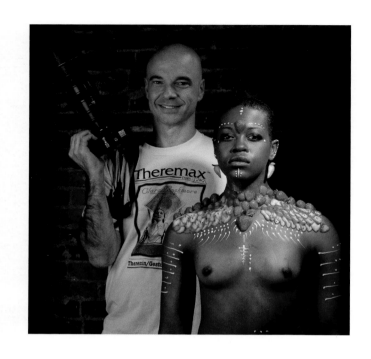

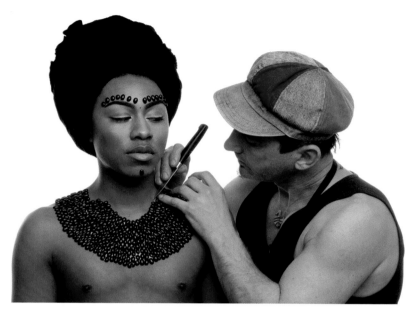

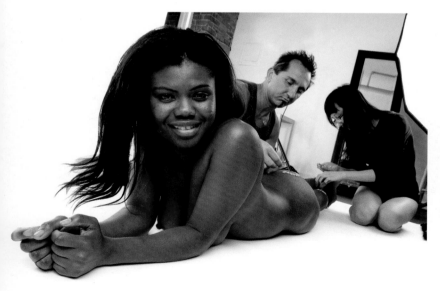

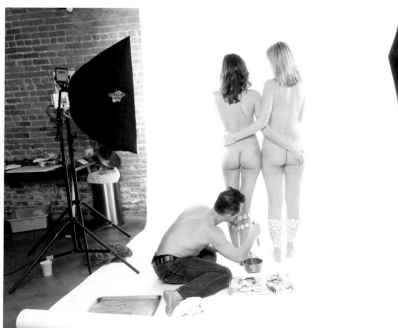

182

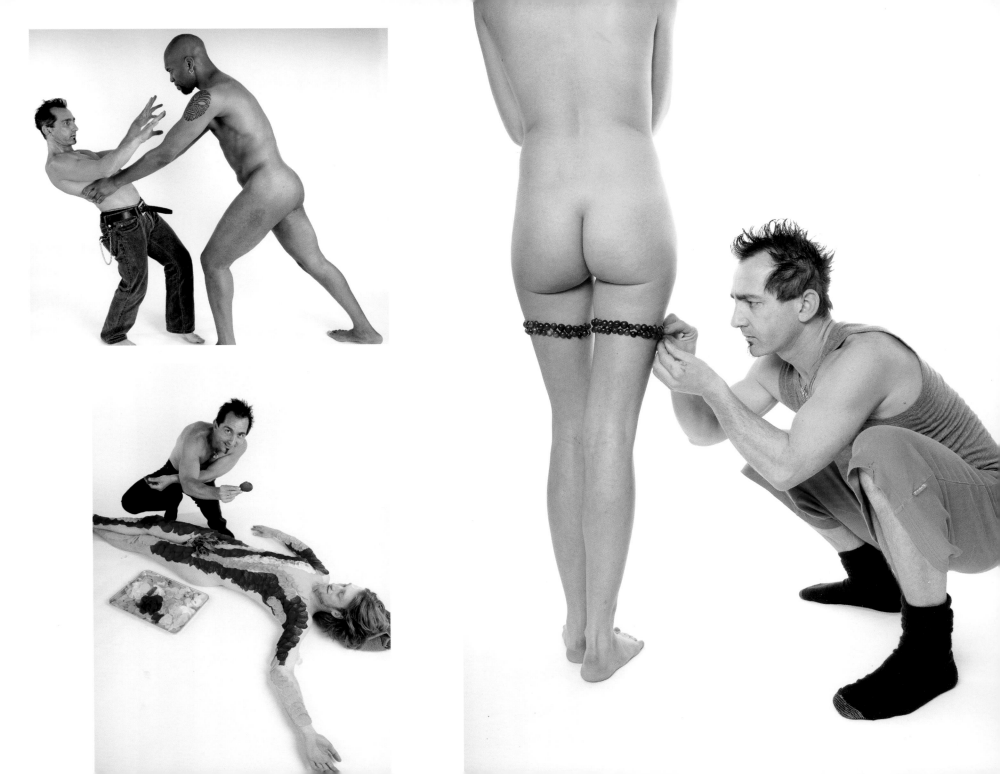

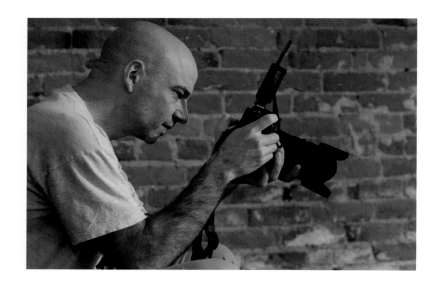

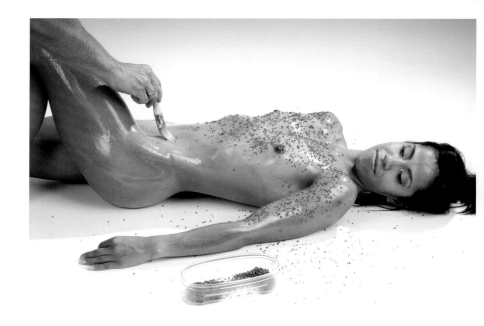

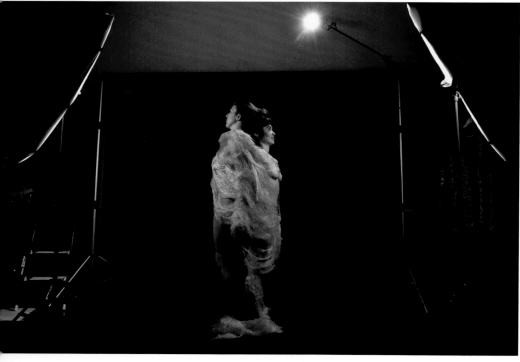

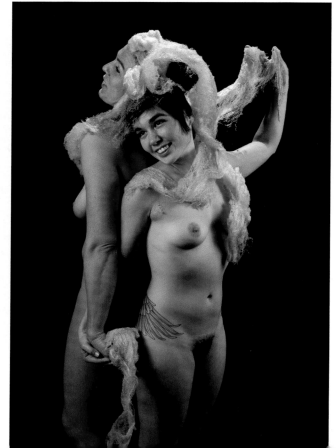

184

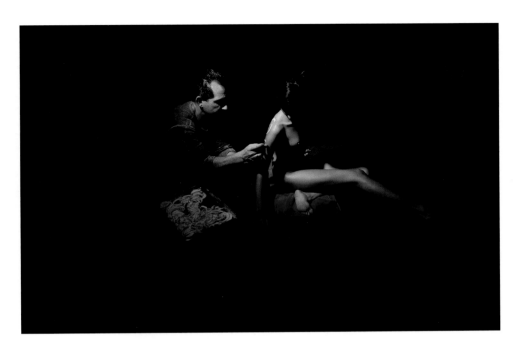

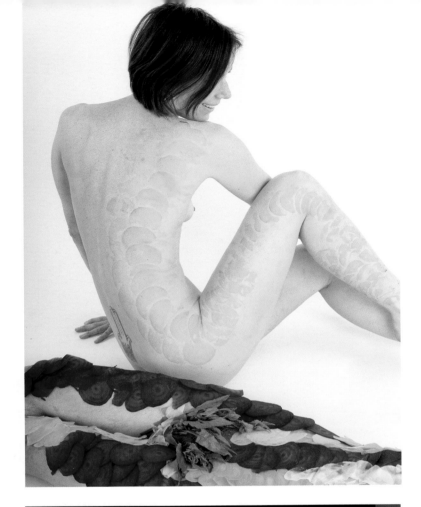

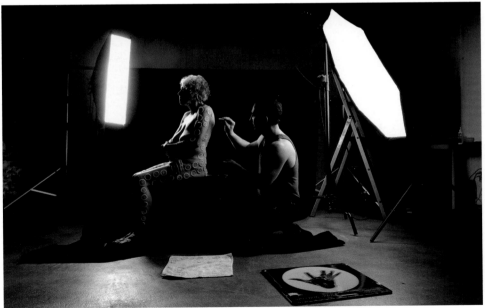

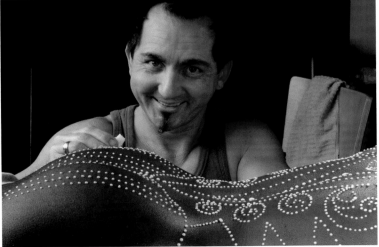

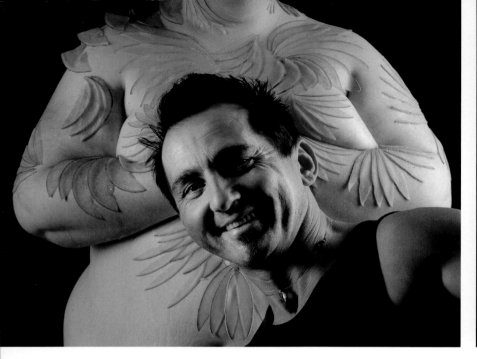

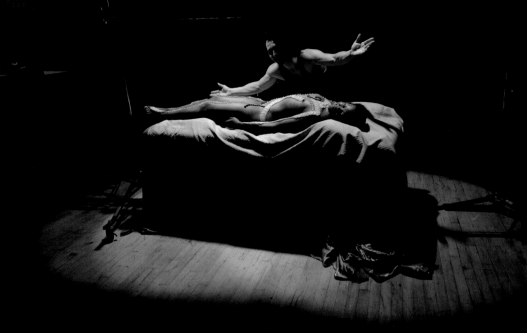

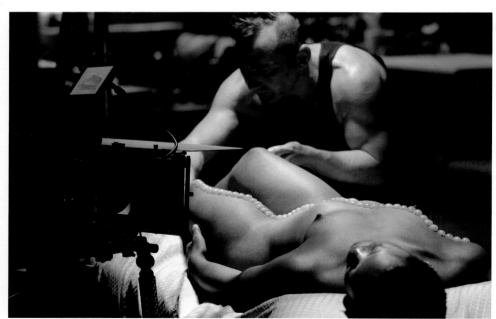

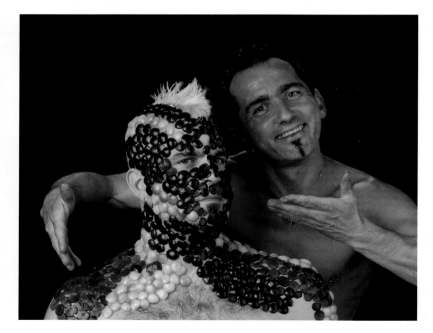

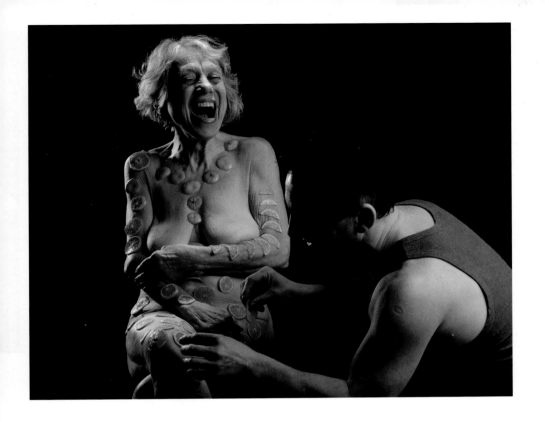

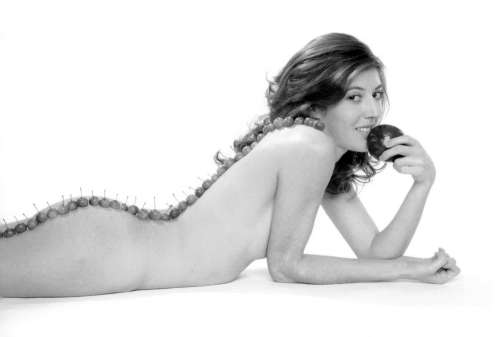

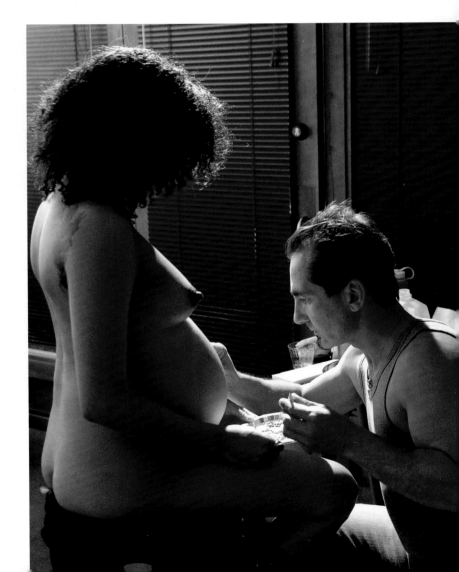

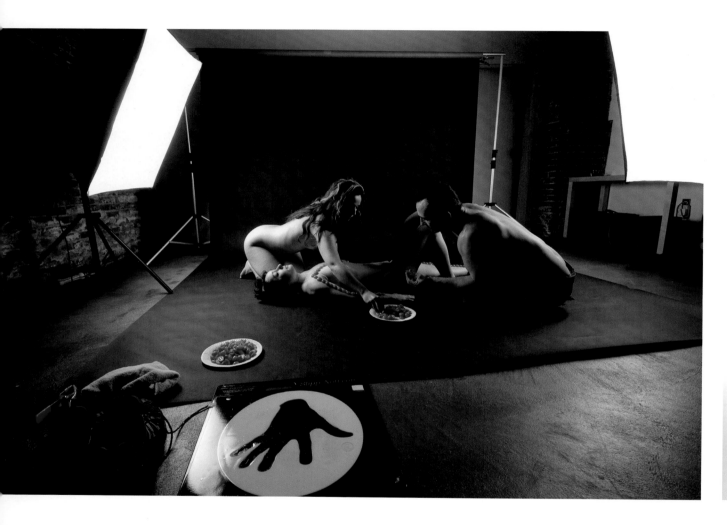
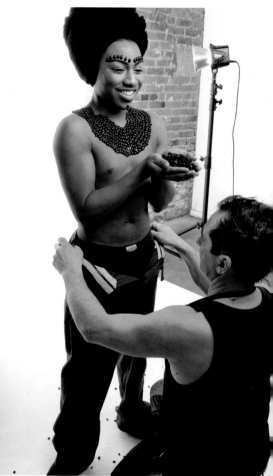

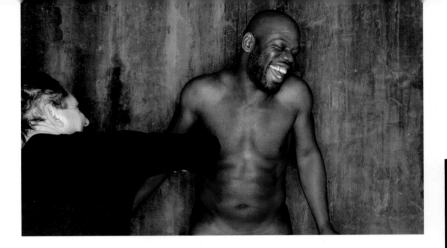
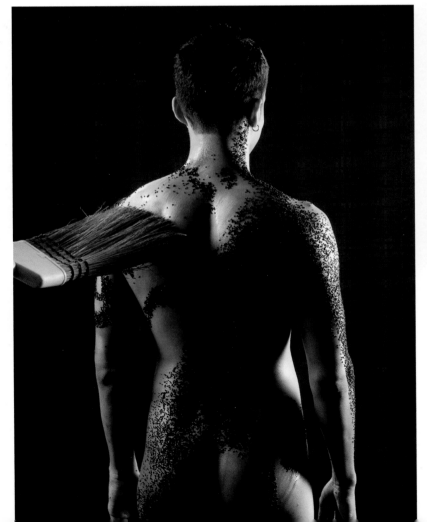
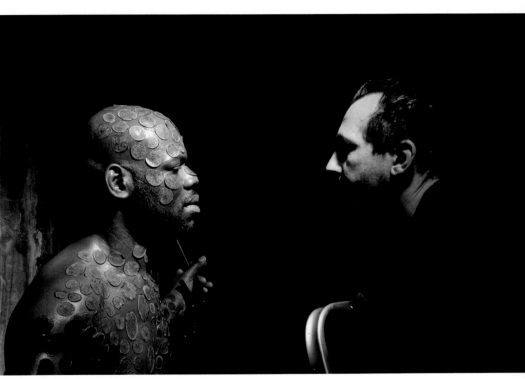

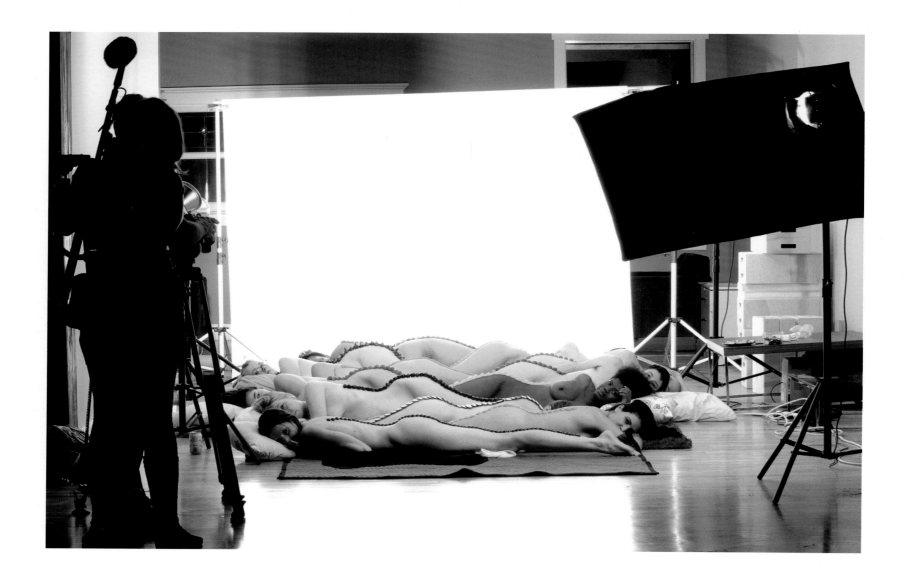

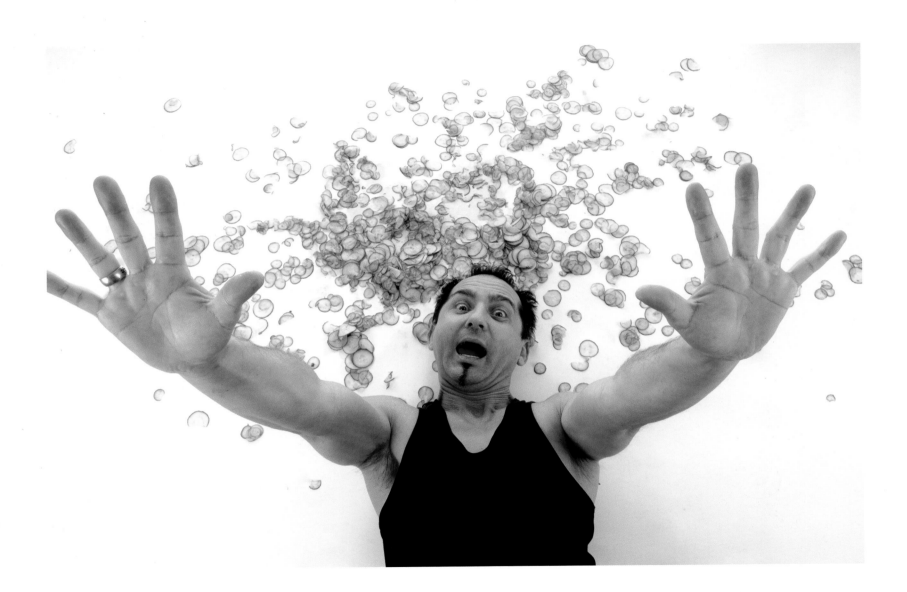

ACKNOWLEDGMENTS

We can't find the words to describe the appreciation we have for all of the amazing people who helped us in so many different ways. *La Figa* would never have been possible without the many, many friends, models, artists, designers, and other supporters who trusted and believed in us as we created this beautiful book. A special thanks goes to Carol Haskins Hetzel for the contribution of her considerable talents towards making *La Figa* a reality.

Thanks, love, and affection from the deepest part of our hearts to…Adraboo, Adriana Medina, Afia Agyei, Alyssa Royse, Amy Trione, Angela King, Beckie Lewis Friend, Brad Younggren, Bri Starkfalla, Bryan Wilkerson, Cayetana San Segundo, Cherry, Clayton Hibbert, Cody Strauss, Dan McComb, Dao Nguyen, Dawn Lake, Dennis Richards, Dog Mountain Farm, E. Theodore Taylor, Elisha Ishii, Ellaina Lewis, Emily O'Neil, Emily Rayson, Eric Wilson, Erin Grabowski, Gabriel Varella, Gaetan Issombo, Georgia Hill, Giannina Silverman, Heather Persinger, Jaclynn "Pinky" Tyler, Jason Wolf, Jen Younggren, Jenée Arthur, Jess Rosa, Joe Pemberton, Jordan Hannah, Joselynn Engstrom, José Luis Rodriguez Guerra, Joy Shumaker, Kristy Friend, Larissa Austin, Leila Anasazi, Lena Ishii, Lisa Copper, Lori Gifford Goodwin, Luc de Montigny, Lucia Mondella, Manita Holtrop, Marcus Trione, Marita Holdaway, Michael Magrath, Michelle Bates, Mina Bast, MK, Monica Day, Nadja Halidmann, Nassim Assefi, Nathan Diehl, Neda Vaseghi, Nishali Nanayakkara, Noah Wheat, Normina Keller, Pafranco, Patricia Ridenour, Perry Emge, Reyna Kammer, Reyshard Elsemaj, Rose Morningstar, Saturnia, Sidney Lewis Friend, Stuart Updegrave, Sue Scharff, Sumit Basu, Terry LaBrue, The Seattle Erotic Art Festival, Tom Haskins, Vanya Vujinovic, Wildflower, and the many others who have helped us along the way.

If you enjoyed *La Figa,* please consider posting a review at your favorite online bookstore.

FOR THE LIST OF INGREDIENTS USED IN THE PHOTOGRAPHS, AS WELL AS LA FIGA NEWS AND EVENTS, BEHIND-THE-SCENES VIDEOS, THE LATEST PHOTOS, RECIPES, AND MUCH MORE, PLEASE VISIT LAFIGAPROJECT.COM.